E. Alexandridis

THE PUPIL

Translated by Terry Telger

With a Foreword by F. C. Blodi

With 35 Figures

Springer-Verlag
New York Berlin Heidelberg Tokyo

E. Alexandridis
Medical Director of the Department
  for Clinical Experimental Ophthalmology
  of the University Eye Clinic
D-6900 Heidelberg, F.R.G.

Library of Congress Cataloging in Publication Data
Alexandridis, Evangelos.
  The pupil.
  Translation of: Die Pupille.
  Includes bibliographies and index.
  1. Ocular manifestations of general diseases.
2. Pupil (Eye)—Examination. 3. Pupil (Eye)—
Effect of drugs on. 4. Iris (Eye)—Diseases. I. Title.
[DNLM: 1. Iris. 2. Iris Diseases. 3. Pupil—drug
effects. 4. Pupil—Physiology. WW 240 A382p]
RE65.A4413 1985   617.7'2   84-26909

Title of Original German Edition: *Die Pupille: Physiologie—*
Untersuchung—Pathologie, Springer-Verlag, Berlin Heidelberg 1982.

Typeset by Bi-Comp Inc., York, Pennsylvania.

9 8 7 6 5 4 3 2 1

ISBN-13: 978-1-4612-9557-0   e-ISBN-13: 978-1-4612-5086-9
DOI: 10.1007/978-1-4612-5086-9

Foreword

This monograph by Professor Alexandridis continues the proud tradition of German ophthalmology in its discussion of the pupil and its importance in the diagnosis of ocular, neurologic, and systemic diseases.

The first encyclopedic work on the pupil was written by Wilbrand and Saenger at the end of the 19th century. This redoubtable pair of physicians collected, analyzed, and classified all the material available at that time, bringing order into the previous chaos.

The second major work was the book by C. v. Behr shortly after World War I. At that time, syphilis had been accurately diagnosed with the aid of serologic tests, and pharmacologic effects on the pupil had become well known.

The third significant development was initiated before World War II by the neurologist Otto Lowenstein, whose work was later brilliantly continued by his pupil and niece Irene Lowenfeld. The introduction of their clinically useful pupillograph made quantitative analysis possible.

There followed a number of important contributions to the knowledge of pupillary physiology and pathology, especially by Harms in Tübingen and Thompson in Iowa City. But the next decisive contribution is this monograph by Alexandridis.

The author has worked for many years on various aspects of the pupil. His portable improved pupillograph (the "Heidelberg" instrument) has made quantitative evaluation easy. Alexandridis could show that dark adaptation, retinal light sensitivity, and many other phenomena could be studied on the basis of the pupillary light reflex. This book contains valuable summaries of the effects of drugs, poisons, and other systemic factors on the pupil.

The chapters on pupillary changes associated with pathologic conditions of the upper visual pathway make fascinating reading.

In addition to pupillography, the author examines less sophisticated but equally important tests, such as pharmacologic reactions and relative afferent defects revealed by the swinging flashlight test.

This book represents an excellent summary of our current knowledge of the physiology and pathology of the pupil. It should be of benefit not only to ophthalmologists and neurologists, but also to internists, neurosurgeons, and psychologists.

F. C. Blodi, M. D.

Preface to the English Edition

The Pupil is intended mainly to aid the practicing ophthalmologist, neurologist, and students of these specialties in the differential diagnosis of pupillary disturbances. In addition, the book gives a concise account of the most recent discoveries relating to the anatomy and physiology of the pupillary pathways.

The idea for this book was suggested by a number of my practicing colleagues, who repeatedly expressed a desire to have a compendium of pupillary abnormalities. I have made every effort to satisfy this demand, both in writing the original book and in preparing the English edition, which is partially revised.

The section on pupillary physiology in Chapter 1, especially as it relates to retinal sensory function, represents a summary of my earlier writings and a monograph published in 1971. Much of the information in Chapters 1 and 2 is presented in a very concise form to serve the immediate needs of the clinician as well as the researcher specializing in the experimental physiology of the pupil.

Chapter 3, which deals with the abnormal pupil, contains a section on pupillary responses to poisonings that will be of interest to a range of specialties.

E. Alexandridis, M.D.

Contents

Contents

CHAPTER 1

The Normal Pupil

I. An Introductory Discussion of Anatomy as It Relates to the Pupil

A. Anatomy of the Iris Musculature

The iris is a disc-shaped diaphragm that is freely suspended within the path of light refraction in the eye. It is perforated by a central opening, the *pupil*, which is shifted slightly toward the nasal side. The main function of the iris is to regulate the amount of light reaching the retina, which it does by constantly adjusting the pupil size. This adjustment is effected by a muscle system composed of a circular part, the sphincter pupillae, and a radial part, the dilator pupillae.

The sphincter pupillae is 0.5–1.0 mm wide and 40–80 μm thick. It consists of bundles of smooth muscle fibers that encircle the pupil in the posterior stroma of the iris, closely approaching the pupillary margin. Firm connecting strands bind the sphincter to surrounding tissues and preserve constriction of the iris even when the muscle is cut, as in a sector iridectomy.

The dilator pupillae is a clear myoepithelial layer, only about 2 μm thick, that extends radially between the sphincter pupillae and ciliary margin. Its posterior surface is covered by the pigment epithelium of the iris (Fig. 1). Both muscles are joined in syncytial fashion by arcade-like connecting strands, which enable each muscle to act directly upon the other. Thus, the sphincter stretches the dilator

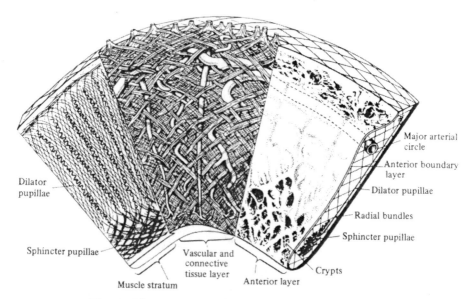

Fig. 1. The structure of the iris. (After Rohen.[232])

while the dilator unfolds the sphincter, with the result that each muscle, on contracting, places its counterpart in an optimum position for initiating its own contraction. The excursion of iris tissue is less at the periphery than at the pupil margin.[221,228,232,233,277]

According to classic theory, both muscles are derived embryologically from the ectodermal portion of the anterior optic cup. However, some authors dispute the ectodermal origin of the iris muscles, especially the dilator, and postulate a mesodermal origin.[102,222,254]

B. Efferent Pathways of the Pupil

The iris muscles are innervated by both sympathetic and parasympathetic pathways. Contrary to classic beliefs, evidence from pupillographic,[164,174,175] electrophysiologic,[28] pharmacologic[91,150,157,244,257] and electron microscopic studies[85] indicates that both the sphincter and the dilator receive sympathetic and parasympathetic fibers, with the sphincter being driven predominantly by the parasympathetic system, and the dilator by the sympathetic.

The parasympathetic innervation of the sphincter pupillae consists of two neurons. Of the entire oculomotor complex, it appears that only the Edinger-Westphal nucleus belongs to the sphincter pupillae. The pathway from this nucleus to the eye is interrupted once by a synapse at the ciliary ganglion (Fig. 2). It is supranuclear inhibition, rather than sympathetic outflow, which causes relaxation of the sphincter during pupillary dilation.[51,164,165]

The sympathetic innervation of the dilator pupillae consists of three neurons. The fibers of the first neuron arise from the hypothalamus and pass to the ciliospinal center located in the lateral part of the anterior horns. From there fibers arise (second neuron) that emerge with the anterior roots and pass to the cervical sympathetic trunk. They then unite with the third neuron in the superior cervical ganglion. From there they travel through the carotid plexus to the first division of the trigeminal nerve, and thence through the long ciliary nerves to the eye (Fig. 3).

C. Afferent Pathway of the Pupillary Light Reflex

The afferent pathway of the pupillary light reflex commences at the retinal photoreceptors, which apparently are identical with the receptors responsible for light perception.[5,7-11,26] Pupillomotor light stimuli are carried to the mesencephalic centers of the sphincter by the optic nerve. The fibers responsible for pupillomotor excitation pass through the optic tract after partially crossing in the chiasm. The afferents separate from the visual fibers in the posterior third of the optic tract and pass the lateral geniculate body on their way to the pretectal area. There they terminate in

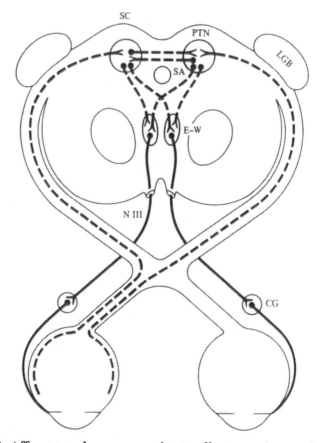

Fig. 2. Afferent and parasympathetic efferent pathway of the pupillary light reflexes. SC, superior colliculus; PTN, pretectal nucleus; LGB, lateral geniculate body; SA, sylvian aqueduct; E-W, Edinger-Westphal nuclei; CG, ciliary ganglion.

the ipsilateral pretectal nucleus. From there the nerve cells send axons in two directions: to the contralateral pretectal nucleus and to the cells of the oculomotor nucleus, with a small number of fibers being distributed to the nucleus on the opposite side (Fig. 2). Thus, the afferent limb of the

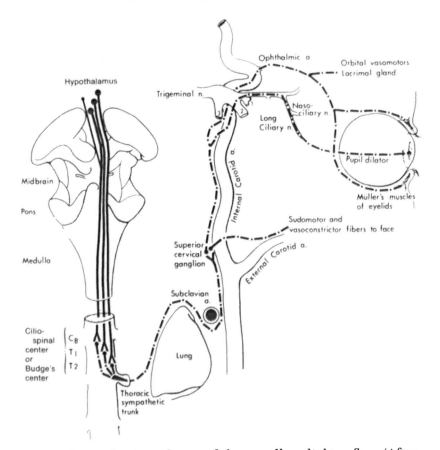

Fig. 3. Sympathetic pathway of the pupillary light reflex. (After Glaser 1978.[108])

pupillary light reflex undergoes a total of three partial crossings before reaching the Edinger-Westphal nuclei.[76] It is unclear whether pupillomotor light stimuli are carried to the pretectal nucleus by collaterals of the optic nerve fibers[39,139] or whether this function is performed by axons arising from special pupillomotor retinal ganglion cells.[2,31,220]

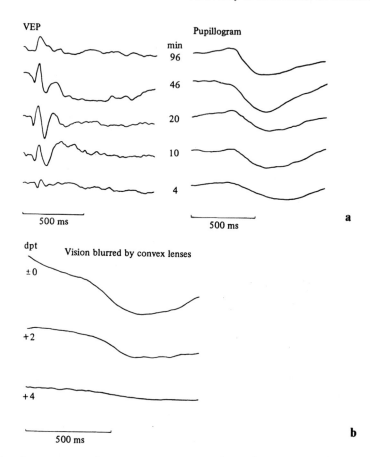

Fig. 4. a: VEP and pupillograms of the human eye obtained under identical conditions in response to alternating geometric patterns. b: Reduction or absence of pupillomotor responses due to refractive error. (After Teping et al.[264])

D. Cortico-Pretectal Connections?

Contrary to classic descriptions, pupilloperimetric studies indicate* that at least a portion of the pupillomotor light impulses pass to the visual cortex before being relayed to

---

* References 19, 72, 122, 124–127, 154, 206, 226, 227, 290.

pupillomotor centers (see Chapter 3, Section II.A.4 for details). The pupillary responses elicited by alternating, geometric visual stimuli also point to the possible existence of cortico-pretectal connections.[253,264,276] Like the visually evoked cortical potential (VECP), pupillomotor responses are decreased or abolished by a refractive error that is sufficient to cause a blurring of vision (Fig. 4). Alternating stimulation of the fovea with monochromatic light of constant intensity also elicits pupillomotor responses.[290]

E. Supranuclear Pathway for the Near-Vision Reflex (Pupillary Synkinesis)

It is known that connections exist between area 19 of the anterior occipital cortex and pupillomotor centers that control the accommodation-convergence synkinesis of the pupil, known also as the near-vision reflex. Electrical stimulation of these areas evokes pupillary constriction, convergence, and accommodation.[37,75,144,189] Whereas light impulses reach the parasympathetic oculomotor nucleus via the pretectal nuclei, cortical impulses for accommodation are carried to the oculomotor nerve outside the pretectal area.[189] The noninvolvement of the pretectal nuclei in accommodation accounts for the clinical signs observed in Argyll Robertson syndrome (see also Chapter 3).

II. Pupil Size

The human pupil ranges in size from 7.5–8 mm at full mydriasis to 1.5–2 mm at full miosis. This means that the area of the pupil (πr^2), and thus the amount of light admitted to the eye, can vary by a factor of 36. At maximum constriction the fibers of the sphincter pupillae are shortened by 87% relative to their length in the resting state,[201] a property possessed by no other smooth muscle in the human body.

A. Variations of Pupil Size

The pupil is small in the first year of life. The dilator pupillae is very poorly developed in the newborn, and even adrenergic drugs produce very little mydriasis at that age. Under normal circumstances the pupil attains its greatest size during adolescence. Women have a larger average pupil size than men, and myopes tend to have larger pupils than emmetropes and hyperopes. In addition, a poorly pigmented (blue) iris will generally have a larger pupil than a heavily pigmented (brown) iris. About 17% of the population have pupils of unequal size (*anisocoria*), but this inequality is pronounced in only about 4%.[195] The degree of the anisocoria is variable. It is seen in normal individuals and can vary in degree from day to day and even hourly. It may coexist in several members of the same family. So far no specific lesions have been demonstrated that could account for this condition. Presumably it is based on an asymmetric

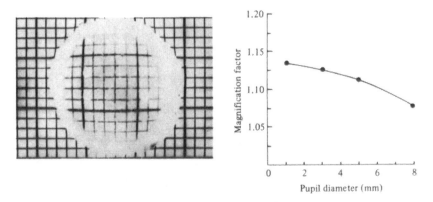

Fig. 5. Apparent enlargement of the human pupil viewed through the cornea and aqueous humor. (After Alexandridis et al.[13])

supranuclear inhibition of the Edinger-Westphal nucleus, which is why the term "simple central anisocoria" is also used.[166] With advancing age the pupils become progressively smaller, and dilation during the dark reflex is much less pronounced than in younger individuals.[46,53,159,167]

B. "Apparent" Pupil Size (Entrance Pupil)

When the eye is examined from the front, the pupil appears slightly magnified as a result of refraction through the anterior chamber. This magnified image is called the "entrance pupil."

The image scale of the entrance pupil is not constant. The magnification of the real pupil to the entrance pupil becomes less pronounced with increasing pupil size due to negative distortion effect from the cornea and aqueous fluid.[13] The image scale is greatest in the paraxial region, and thus when the pupil is constricted. On average the entrance pupil of the human eye appears to be magnified by a factor of 1.13 (in extreme miosis) to 1.08 (in extreme mydriasis) (Fig. 5). Actual pupil size can be measured with the aid of a fundus or gonioscopic contact lens applied to the surface of the eye.

III. Pharmacologic Effects on the Pupil

Pupil-active agents are autonomic drugs that affect the pupil by altering either the sympathetic innervation of the dilator pupillae or the parasympathetic innervation of the pupillary sphincter. In both the sympathetic and parasympathetic systems, the transmission of efferent impulses from the pre- to the postganglionic neuron is mediated by acetylcholine. At postganglionic junctions the transmitter substances vary, with norepinephrine being released at the nerve endings of the sympathetic neuron and acetylcholine at the nerve endings of the parasympathetic (Fig. 6). The terms adrenergic and cholinergic are commonly used to characterize the actions of pharmacologic agents. Thus, a cholinergic agent produces an effect similar to that associated with the liberation of acetylcholine from the nerves, whereas an adrenergic agent mimics the effect of norepinephrine release.

A. Locally Administered Pupil-Active Agents

1. Adrenergic Agents

The local adrenergic agents most commonly used in ophthalmology are epinephrine (adrenaline), phenylephrine (Neosynephrine), tyramine, and cocaine. The first two agents are direct adrenergics, i.e., they interact directly with the receptor in the muscle and behave like the physiologic

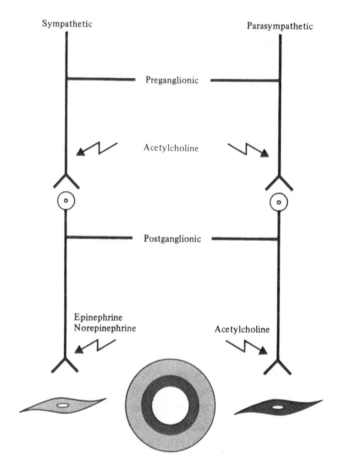

Fig. 6. Pre- and postganglionic transmitter substances of the sympathetic and parasympathetic nervous systems.

transmitter substance norepinephrine. Tyramine and cocaine are indirect adrenergics. Tyramine liberates norepinephrine from the sympathetic nerve ending, whereas cocaine enhances the effect of endogenous norepinephrine by preventing its inactivation through rebinding at nerve terminals.

Another indirect adrenergic is ephedrine, which currently is marketed only as a combination product. Its mode

TABLE 1. Locally Administered Pupil-Active Adrenergic Agents

Direct adrenergics	
Epinephrine (Adrenaline) Phenylephrine (Neosynephrine)	} React directly with the muscle receptor
Indirect adrenergics	
Cocaine	Enhances the effect of norepinephrine
Tyramine Ephedrine Hydroxyamphetamine (Paredrine)	} Liberate stored norepinephrine

of action is similar to that of tyramine. Hydroxyamphetamine (Paredrine) is also included in the class of indirect adrenergics (Table 1).

2. Antiadrenergic Agents

A number of drugs produce miosis by blocking sympathetic transmission. An example is guanethidine (Ismelin), which has been used in drop form for the treatment of glaucoma and to prevent lid retraction in thyrotoxicosis. It interferes with the capacity of sympathetic terminals to store epinephrine, thus creating a neurotransmitter deficit that lessens response to sympathetic outflow. Thymoxamine, an α-blocking drug, is also used to induce miosis or to abolish the mydriatic effect of direct adrenergics.[45]

Prostaglandin, which is produced ubiquitously in tissues, including the iris, probably also causes miosis through an antiadrenergic effect.[94] Aspirin and indomethacin inhibit prostaglandin synthesis. This underlies the value of indomethacin in cataract surgery as a means of preventing prostaglandin-induced miosis.[153]

TABLE 2. Locally Administered Pupil-Active Cholinergic
Agents

Direct cholinergics	
Pilocarpine	
Carbachol	} React directly with the muscle receptor
Mecholyl	
Indirect cholinergics	
Physostigmine	
(Eserine)	
Prostigmine	
Mintacol	} Inhibit cholinesterase
DFP	
Demecarium bromide	
(Tosmilene)	

3. Cholinergic Agents

Cholinergic agents act like acetylcholine to produce a parasympathomimetic miosis. The principal local cholinergics are pilocarpine, carbachol, mecholyl, physostigmine (Eserine), prostigmine, mintacol, DFP, and demecarium bromide (Tosmilene). Pilocarpine, carbachol, and mecholyl are direct cholinergics, meaning that they react directly with the target organ receptor. The remaining substances are indirect cholinergics. They act by blocking or destroying cholinesterase (cholinesterase inhibitors), thereby slowing the degradation of acetylcholine and increasing its miotic effect (Table 2).

TABLE 3. Locally Administered
Pupil-Active Anticholinergic Agents

Atropine	
Scopolamine	
Homatropine	} Block the muscle receptor
Cyclopentolate	
Tropicamide	

4. Anticholinergic Agents

The most important agents that block parasympathetic transmission at nerve endings are atropine, scopolamine, homatropine, cyclopentolate, and tropicamide. These agents bind to the target-organ receptor site without reacting with it (Table 3), thereby blocking the action of acetylcholine (anticholinergic effect).

IV. Reflex Changes in the Pupil

A. Pupillary Unrest (Pupillary Oscillations)

The iris continuously adjusts the pupil size in an effort to maintain a constant level of retinal illumination. This function of the iris is not a simple reflex, but is the result of a true regulatory process.

A closed-loop servomechanism regulates the amount of light admitted to the eye.[49,88,259,260] The sensor for this servomechanism is the retina. The mydriatic and miotic centers represent the servomotor, while the iris serves as the effector (Fig. 7). A change in the intensity of retinal illumination leads to a change in the flow of impulses to the pupillomotor centers that adjust pupil size. This is accompanied by a concurrent change in the sensitivity of the retina (sensor). This change, combined with a reduction of retinal illumination by pupillary constriction, initiates a new change in pupillomotor outflow, and so on. Constant pupillary unrest, which is particularly marked under conditions of light adaptation, is a byproduct of the function of this servomechanism—an expression of an ongoing process in which retinal illumination is adjusted to an "ideal" value.[278] There is evidence that both the respiratory rate and the blood pulsation rate also contribute to pupillary unrest. The origin of other periodic fluctuations of pupil size at frequencies of 1/10 Hz and 1/3 Hz remains unclear.[81] The frequency of the pupil-

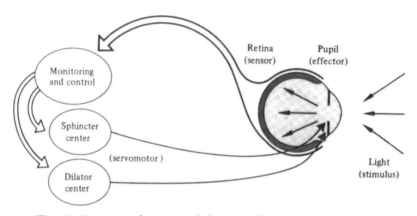

Fig. 7. Servomechanism of the pupillary light response.

lary oscillations is approximately 3 Hz in the healthy adult, even when light intensity is varied in sine-wave fashion. The cause of this relatively low frequency is the smooth musculature of the iris. Like all other iris functions,[155,203] the frequency of pupillary oscillations decreases markedly with age,[21] probably due to sclerosis of the iris blood vessels and degeneration of the iris stroma and iris musculature.[233]

B. Pupillary Responses to Light

When light is presented to one eye only, the pupil of the nonstimulated eye will also contract. This phenomenon is called the *consensual pupillary light reflex*. The bilaterality of the reflex derives from the fact that each retina has connections with both optic tracts, and each tract with both oculomotor nuclei. The pupillary reaction will vary depending on the duration of the light stimulus.

1. Pupillary Response to a Sustained Light Stimulus: The Tonic Light Reflex

If steady illumination is presented to the eye, the pupil will undergo large initial oscillations followed by a gradual sta-

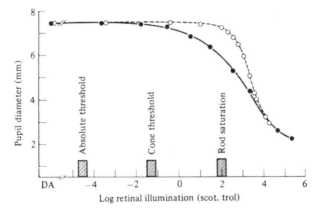

Fig. 8. Size of the human pupil as a function of retinal illumination. -•-, Illumination with white light; -o-, illumination with monochromatic light (486 nm). Adaptation field 160°. (After Alexandridis et al.[17])

bilization of size in what is termed the *tonic pupillary light reflex*. At higher light intensities the pupil becomes progressively smaller as it oscillates, whereas at low light intensities the final pupil size is larger than that noted at the start of illumination. When a dark-adapted eye is illuminated at levels that are subthreshold for the cone receptors, there is an initial, momentary constriction of the pupil followed by a redilation to the initial size ("pupillary escape"). There is evidence that the mechanisms responsible for this response reside both in the retina and in the pretectal nuclei.[261] Constriction of the pupil in the presence of sustained illumination (Fig. 8) commences at luminance levels corresponding to the range of photopic (day) vision.[17,256] When the eyes are illuminated with monochromatic light, pupil constriction begins at luminance values at which the sensitivity of the rod mechanism begins to fall off.[4] When circumscribed portions of the retina are illuminated, the light striking the fovea will be the main determinant of the pupillary response.[55] Like cone sensitivity, pupil size varies with the angle of light incidence.[25,256] In rod monochromasia, or failure of photopic function, the pupil remains markedly larger than normal.[6,9,15] On the other hand, in Oguchi's disease, or failure of rod function, the pupillary response to sustained light is identical to that in the normal eye.[86]

All these findings suggest that the principal "sensor" for the pupillary response to sustained light is the photopic system of the retina.

2. Dependence of Visual Acuity on Pupil Size

In the emmetropic eye the pupil assumes the size that is necessary for optimum sharpness of vision.[66] When uncorrected ametropia exists, visual acuity shows a pronounced dependence on pupil size, the degree of this dependence increasing with the degree of the refractive error.[33,34]

3. Pupillary Response to Darkness

The withdrawal of light from the light-adapted eye causes the pupil to dilate in two phases: a rapid initial phase followed by a second, relatively gradual dilatory phase.[140] The course of this dark response depends on the magnitude and duration of the previous light adaptation.[52] The rapid phase of the dark response occurs during the first 10–30 s after light is withdrawn. The definitive pupil size is attained within 4–6 min, depending on prior light adaptation. This period corresponds to the amount of time required to increase the sensitivity of the photopic system during dark adaptation. This fact, and the disturbance of pupillary dilation during dark adaptation that occurs in rod monochromasia,[6,9,15,90] suggest that the photopic system of the retina plays a key sensing role in the mechanism controlling the dark response.

4. Pupillary Response to a Single, Brief Light Stimulus: The Phasic Light Reflex

Illumination of the retina by a brief light stimulus (light flash) triggers the production of a correspondingly short pupillomotor impulse. Because the stimulus is transitory, the resulting pupillary constriction is followed by redilation. This response is called the *phasic light reflex* of the pupil. Like the tonic light reflex, the phasic reflex is consensual in man and higher mammals, i.e., both eyes react when only one eye is stimulated. The simultaneous stimulation of both eyes elicits a stronger pupil constriction for a given light intensity than does unilateral stimulation.[223] Both retinal receptor systems act as sensors for the phasic light reflex, with the prevailing adaptation state determining whether the rod or cone mechanism will control the reflex. The phasic light reflex is dependent on the luminance, duration, and wavelength of the light stimulus, as well as on the adaptation state of the retina.[1,5,7,8,10–12,55,88,176] The spectral sensitivity of the phasic light reflex (Fig. 9) is virtually identical to the scotopic and photopic sensitivity curve obtained by psychophysical measurement.[17,26] Even in persons with defective color vision, pupillomotor response parallels sensory response in the disturbed region of the spectrum.[184] On the other hand, failure of the rod mechanism in retinitis pigmentosa does not alter the behavior of the phasic pupillary reflex during light adaptation.[22]

a. Latent Period of the Pupillary Light Reflex

The time elapsing between the presentation of a light stimulus and the onset of iris contraction is called the *latent period* of the pupillary light reflex. It, too, depends on the luminance, duration, and wavelength of the light stimulus and on the adaptation state of the retina.[11,55,88,176] The shortest latent period for this reflex in the normal eye is between 0.2 and 0.25 s; the longest is from 0.4 to 0.5 s.

b. The Pupil on Lid Closure

In bright light a small pupillary light reflex is observed each time the eyelids are closed and reopened. This reflex does

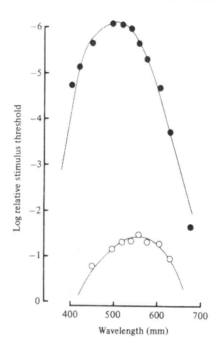

Fig. 9. Scotopic (-●-) and photopic (-○-) spectral sensitivity of the human eye as determined from pupillary light reflexes. (After Alexandridis et al.[17])

not occur in darkness.[7,279] It may be assumed, therefore, that brief lid closure produces a slight but definite increase in retinal sensitivity.

C. Accommodation-Convergence Synkinesis

The response to near vision, i.e., accommodation of the lenses and convergence of the eyes, is accompanied by pupillary constriction. This is not a reflex, but rather an associated movement or *synkinesis* involving a triad of events. These events are controlled and coordinated by supranuclear pathways. Accommodation, convergence, and miosis can be elicited, either in association or in isolation, by electrical stimulation of areas 19 and 22 of the anterior occipital cortex.[144] The cortical impulses necessary for accommodation-convergence synkinesis are carried by appropriate fibers either directly or indirectly through the visual association fields to the superior colliculi, and from there to the caudal portions of the oculomotor nuclei. The pretectal nuclei, though important centers of the light reflex system, are not involved in accommodation-convergence synkinesis.[75,189] When convergence without accommodation is induced by having subjects view distant objects through prisms, the resulting pupillary constriction[225] is identical to that which accompanies accommodation without convergence.[184,185]

D. The Pupil in Sleep

Pupil size, like so many other physiologic processes, parallels the level of consciousness. Thus, as sleep approaches, the pupil becomes smaller. During sleep both the active sympathetic innervation of the dilator and the inhibition of the oculomotor nucleus are diminished, placing the pupil in a miotic state.[165,171,289]

E. Psychosensory Reflex Dilation of the Pupil

Emotional states such as anxiety, fear, joy, and surprise cause the pupil to dilate. Normal light reflexes remain disturbed as long as the dilation progresses under the influence of the emotional excitement.[104,178] Especially in young persons, strong physical and emotional stimuli can suppress the pupillary light reflex.[279] Loud noises also cause dilation of the pupil. States of heightened central nervous system arousal as well as sensory, psychic, emotional, and intellectual stimuli enlarge the pupil by simultaneously activating two nervous mechanisms: adrenergic innervation of the dilator pupillae, causing this muscle to contract, and passive elongation of the sphincter pupillae through the inhibition of parasympathetic discharges from the oculomotor nucleus. Pain stimulates mydriasis in a similar fashion.[30,174]

F. Stimulation of the Vestibular Apparatus

Stimulation of the vestibular apparatus leads to pupillary dilation. This is attributed to the fact that a portion of the sympathetic fibers which supply the iris musculature traverse the middle ear. This would account for the dilator paresis that sometimes occurs following mastoid surgery.[201]

G. The Orbicularis Phenomenon

Closure of the eyelid causes the pupil to constrict. This is especially marked during forceful lid closure and thus during strong activation of the orbicularis muscle. This phenomenon is not a reflex, but an associated movement (synkinesis). It is considered evidence of a direct connection between the facial nerve nucleus and the cells of the oculomotor nucleus that supply the superior rectus and obliquus inferior muscles.[201] The miosis is most conspicuous when the eyelids are forcibly help open while the patient attempts to close them.

H. The Trigeminal Reflex

Irritation of the eyelids, conjunctiva, or cornea elicits a brief dilation of the pupil followed by constriction. The initial mydriasis is a pain response. The subsequent miosis is bilateral but is more pronounced in the pupil on the affected side.[201]

CHAPTER 2

Examination of the Pupil

I. Methods and Instrumentation

A. Methods of Direct Observation

1. Assessment of Pupil Size

Methods of direct observation are best for routine assessments of pupil size. In the past a variety of devices have been utilized to measure pupil size by comparison with standard patterns or scales,[62,245,270] or, for a more accurate assessment, by microscopic inspection.[240,246]

The simplest device is the Haab scale, on which are printed a series of black circles, graduated in size, that are compared with the subject's pupil. Held against the temporal area next to the eye, the scale is kept out of the subject's line of vision so that accommodation effects are avoided (Fig. 10). Pupil size can be determined to an accuracy of ±0.2 mm. The main disadvantage of this method is the inability to evaluate pupil size in darkness.

2. Testing the Phasic Light Reflex

In both the office and hospital settings, routine assessments of pupillary light reflexes traditionally have been based on direct observations of the pupillary state. The advantage of

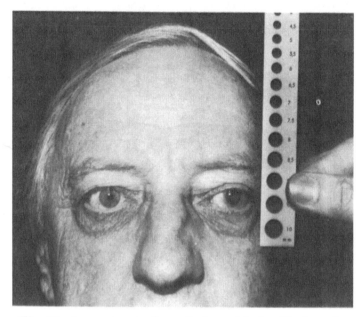

Fig. 10. Assessment of pupil size with the Haab scale.

direct observation is the ease and rapidity with which results are obtained (cf. Marcus Gunn phenomenon, swinging flashlight test, etc., Chapter 3, Section II.B). The classic "differential pupillometer"[138] and "pupillomotor perimeter"[100] relied on direct observation with a magnifying loupe to evaluate the pupillary state.

B. Entoptic Methods

Entoptic methods are based on a subjective self-assessment of pupil size (Fig. 11). A number of techniques using this principle have been developed and described.[55,163,180] Bouma states that these methods are accurate to about 0.1 mm. Like other methods of direct observation, the entoptic

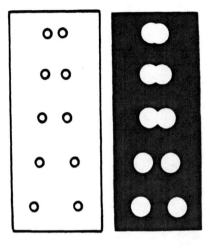

Fig. 11. Principle of entoptic pupillometry. Two small holes on a card held close to the cornea appear to the eye as circles. When the circles appear to touch each other, the distance between the holes in that pair will be equal to the diameter of the pupil. (After Cogan.[73])

methods do not enable a direct assessment of pupillary responses in darkness.

C. Photographic Methods of Examination

Sequential photographs of the pupil provide a useful means of monitoring the pupillary state over a designated interval of time (Fig. 12). By using infrared-sensitive film, one can record pupil size even in total darkness without affecting the adaptation of the eye.[5,83,101,172,182,216] The disadvantages of this method are its limited temporal resolution, the long time needed to evaluate photographic records, and the high cost of infrared film. Photographic methods include the various techniques of kymography,[23,42,70,214] in which a continuous film record of a narrow, central pupillary zone is made through a slitlike aperture (Fig. 13).

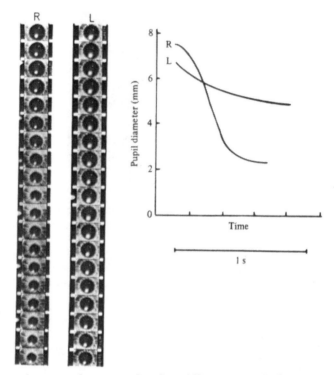

Fig. 12. Photographic records of pupillary states and the resulting pupillograms.

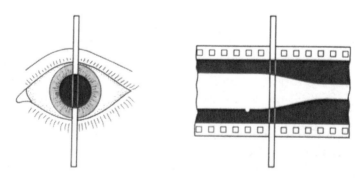

Fig. 13. A kymogram is a continuous photographic record made through a slitlike aperture, showing the state of a narrow, central pupillary zone.

D. Infrared Reflex Pupillography: The Heidelberg Pupillograph

Pupillography provides a continuous record of the phasic light reflex of the pupil. The technique is based on the principle of infrared reflex photometry.[78,88,188] The portable infrared reflex pupillograph (Heidelberg pupillograph) was developed for routine clinical assessments of the pupillary light reflex.[7,18] A narrow beam of infrared light is shined into the eye through a circular orifice in a photoelectric cell. The light reflected back from the eye (chiefly the iris) strikes the photoelectric cell located about 3 cm from the ocular surface, and its intensity is displayed on an oscillograph (Fig. 14). Because the fundus of the eye reflects only 1–2% of incident infrared radiation,[259,260] the deflections on the oscil-

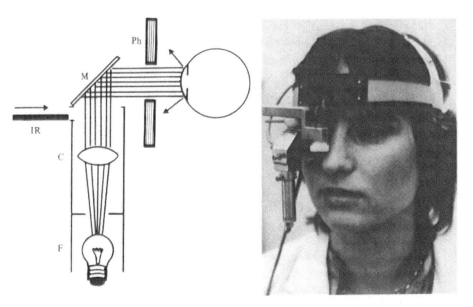

Fig. 14. Schematic diagram of the Heidelberg pupillograph, and its appearance when in use. Ph, Silicon photoelectric cell; M, semitransparent mirror; IR, infrared filter; C, condenser; F, filament lamp. (From Alexandridis et al.[18])

lograph produced by changes in the photoelectric current represent changes in the area of the iris, rather than the pupil. With this scaled-down portable model, one can obtain pupillographic records without immobilizing the patient's head, since the photoelectric cell maintains a fixed distance and position relative to the eye. With its virtually unlimited resolving power, this method is ideal for analyzing the temporal characteristics of the pupillary light reflexes, such as the latent period. The disadvantage of the method is its inability to determine absolute pupil size. A contact lens pupillograph operating on the same principle has recently been described.[61]

E. Electrode Scanning of the Eye (Television Pupillometry)

This technique was introduced by Lowenstein et al.[177] and has since been widely used in numerous variations.[32,106,194,239] A television camera, usually infrared-sensitive, is used to transmit an image of the anterior portion of the eye to a monitor screen. Then parameters of pupillary function such as the phasic light reflex (pupillogram), the amplitude of the light reflex, etc. can be continuously evaluated using various image analysis techniques (Fig. 15). The disadvantage of this method is its poor temporal resolution compared with infrared reflex pupillography.

F. The Pupillogram

A continuous record of the phasic pupillary light reflex, called a *pupillogram*, is shown in Fig. 16. The record pictured is an infrared reflex pupillogram. It can be seen that the area of the iris first increases rapidly and then more slowly as the reflex progresses (indicated by a downward deflection of the curve). After attaining a maximum, the iris area begins to decrease—rapidly at first, as before, and then more slowly—as the pupil redilates to its original size.

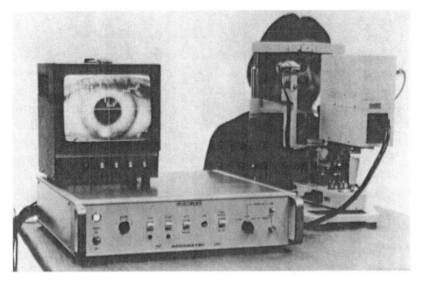

Fig. 15. Television pupillometer with facilities for image analysis.

1. Quantitative Evaluation of the Pupillogram

Pupillary redilation takes place at a slower rate than constriction. The difference between the constriction time and redilation time depends on the intensity of the light stimulus. The stronger the retinal stimulation, the greater the

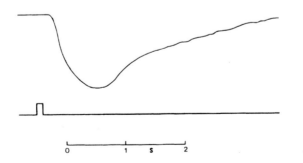

Fig. 16. Pupillogram of the human eye. IR reflexometric record obtained with a light-flash stimulus (0.1 s).

difference. The intraindividual variability of this difference is very large.

The time from the onset of pupillary constriction to maximum iris contraction, called the *peak time*, ranges between 0.15 and 1.2 s. Pupillary redilation, measured from the point of maximum iris contraction to the recovery of initial pupil size, ranges from 0.4 to 5.0 s, depending on the factors noted above.[88]

If we wish to evaluate the phasic light reflex quantitatively, we can use the pupillogram to determine the following parameters:

The amplitude or magnitude of the reflex change in iris area following light stimulation

The latency of the light reflex, i.e., the interval between the start of the light stimulus and the onset of the reflex change in iris area

The light energy required for a constant amplitude

The pupillomotor threshold, i.e., the smallest amount of light that can elicit a pupillary response.

II. Pupillary Light Reflexes in the Evaluation of Retinal Function

A. Evaluation of Normal Retinal Function

The pupillary light reflexes depend on the adaptation state of the retina,[10] the intensity and wavelength of the light stimulus,[17,26,249] and the magnitude and duration of the light stimulus.[8] Thus, the pupillary reactions to light provide an objective means for evaluating the sensory function of the retina. By measuring the pupillomotor threshold at short intervals during dark adaptation, it is possible to construct a dark adaptation curve using the pupillographic method (Fig. 17). The spectral sensitivity of the retina can also be evaluated objectively by determining the pupillary response thresholds to stimulation with monochromatic light (Fig. 9). Depending on the retinal adaptation state, this sensitivity will correspond to that measured subjectively.

B. Evaluation of Abnormal Retinal Function

Like the physiologic suppression of a retinal receptor system by adaptation processes, the morbid failure of a receptor system can be demonstrated objectively by changes in pupillary light reactions. In rod monochromasia, for example, the spectral distribution of pupillomotor sensitivity corresponds in all adaptation states to the scotopic (rod) sensitivity curve.[9] In individuals with defects of color vision, a

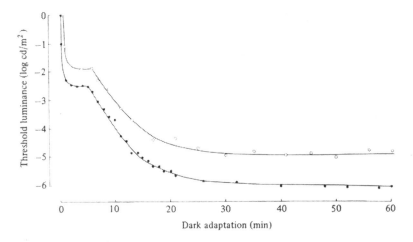

Fig. 17. Dark adaptation curve of the human eye as determined from pupillary light reflexes (*open circles*) and subjectively (*filled circles*). (After Alexandridis.[10])

parallel response is observed between sensory function and pupillomotor function in the disturbed region of the spectrum.[134] In patients with hereditary pigmentary degeneration of the retina, pupillomotor sensitivity corresponds to the sensitivity of the receptors whose function is still intact. In patients with night blindness, it is identical to the sensitivity of the photopic system despite dark adaptation.[22]

C. Objective Perimetry

Pupillary light reflexes can be used to document subjective complaints. The principle of objective perimetry was first described by Harms,[124] and the method was later shown to be valid at the receptor level.[10,57,173,249] Pupillographic perimetry is best performed using techniques of infrared reflex photometry or infrared television image analysis. The examiner shines a narrow beam of light onto small, circumscribed areas of the retina along a meridian and then notes the light intensity at which the first recordable pupillomotor response is elicited (the "pupillomotor threshold"). The pro-

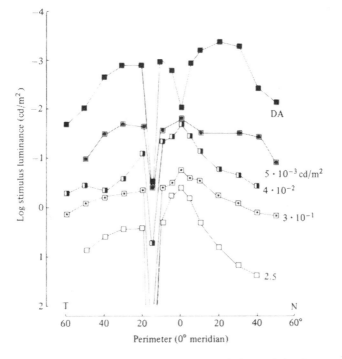

Fig. 18. Profile of the pupillomotor excitability of the human retina for various adaptation states along the 0° meridian. Adaptation luminance is indicated next to each curve. (After Alexandridis.[10])

file of the pupillomotor excitability of the retina obtained in this way resembles the profile of light perception obtained under identical conditions. During dark adaptation, pupillomotor excitability is higher at the periphery than in the macular area. During light adaptation, on the other hand, sensitivity is greatest over the macula.[10] The interval between pupillomotor excitation and light perception depends on the adaptation state of the retina as well as on the size of the area stimulated and the duration of the stimulus.[8] Under all adaptation conditions the "blind spot" can be demonstrated by stimulating an area of appropriate size and recording the pupillomotor response (Fig. 18). To date, pupillographic pe-

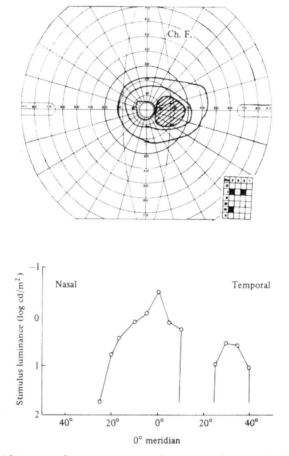

Fig. 19. Objective demonstration of a reported visual field loss and of an enlarged blind spot (**top,** optic atrophy) utilizing pupillary light reflexes.

rimetry has proved to be of great clinical value as a critical simulation test. All reported visual field losses up to a range of about 50° from the macula (Fig. 19) can be demonstrated objectively by this method.

CHAPTER 3

The Abnormal Pupil

I. Irregularities of the Pupil

The normal pupil is shifted slightly toward the nasal side of the cornea, and a slight deviation from roundness is not uncommon. Significant irregularities of the pupil can have numerous causes and should be excluded before pupillary reactions are tested.

A. Malformations and Anomalies of the Iris

1. Corectopia

The pupil is displaced in various directions, usually nasally and inferiorly, and is noncircular (Fig. 20). Frequently the displacement is bilateral and symmetric.

2. Microcoria

This is a very rare condition in which the dilator pupillae is absent, resulting in an extreme congenital miosis.

3. Colobomas

Colobomas may occur alone or in association with other ocular malformations. They most commonly involve the inferior nasal portion of the iris and are wider at the pupillary margin than at the iris root.[208]

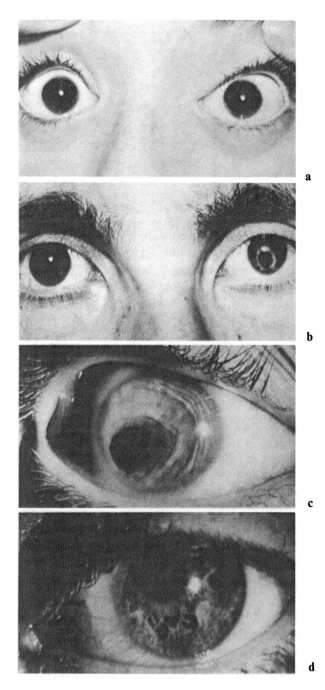

a

b

c

d

4. Congenital Aniridia

Congenital absence of the iris is usually bilateral and is often accompanied by secondary glaucoma. The iris is rudimentary and is visible only with a gonioscope. Aniridia is frequently associated with Wilms' tumor and skeletal malformations.[197,236]

5. Persistent Pupillary Membrane

A persistent pupillary membrane is not an uncommon finding during slit-lamp examinations. Sometimes the membrane is visible with the unaided eye. It may coexist with other ocular malformations.[69]

B. Progressive Essential Iris Atrophy

The main feature of this disease is atrophy of the iris stroma, leading to pupillary distortion and ectopia (Fig. 21). The patient develops a secondary angle-closure glaucoma that is refractory to treatment.[77]

Systemic diseases such as Rieger's syndrome and xeroderma pigmentosum can produce similar changes.[24,77,160]

In Labrador, a severe atrophy of the sphincter pupillae, presumably hereditary, resulting in a distortion of pupillary shape is a very common affliction in persons of European origin.[54]

C. Trauma

Contusions of the eyeball can produce various types of iris injury that are associated with pupil irregularities.

◁ **Fig. 20. a–d:** Corectopia. The pupils are displaced (a) nasally and inferiorly, **(b)** inferiorly with anisocoria, **(c)** temporally and inferiorly, **(d)** nasally and superiorly.

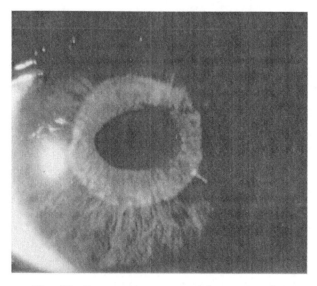

Fig. 21. Progressive essential iris atrophy.

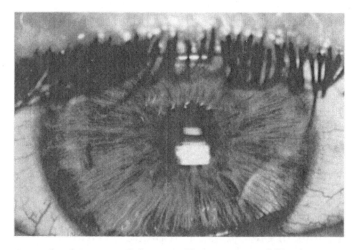

Fig. 22. Multiple tears of the pupillary margin following a contusion of the globe.

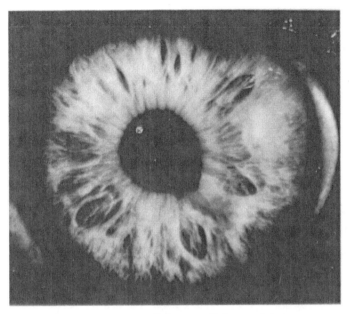

Fig. 23. Distortion of the pupil by an iris tumor.

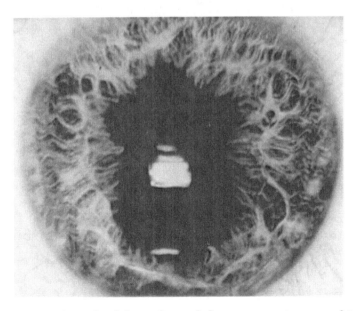

Fig. 24. Cloverleaf-shaped pupil due to posterior synechiae.

1. Tears of the Pupillary Margin and Sphincter

These may be single or multiple (Fig. 22). Traumatic mydriasis and a loss or disturbance of pupillary light reflexes
are frequently permanent. In other cases the pupil may re-
cover its function despite multiple sphincter lacerations.

2. Iridodialysis

A small iridodialysis (iris root avulsion) produces a characteristic D-shaped distortion of the pupil. The reactivity of
the iris is most noticeably disturbed in the pupillary sector
with the greatest radius. A large iridodialysis creates a dou-
ble pupil, resulting in monocular diplopia.

3. Traumatic Aniridia

Complete absence of the iris following trauma is the result
of a circumferential iris root avulsion, sometimes associated
with a rupture of the limbus.

D. Tumors of the Iris

Tumors of the iris stroma lead to ectropion uveae and an
irregularly shaped pupil (Fig. 23).

E. Inflammatory Diseases of the Iris

An irregular pupil in the setting of iritis is due to the presence of posterior synechiae (Fig. 24). The reactivity of the
iris is correspondingly diminished.

II. Pupillary Disturbances Accompanying Neuroophthalmologic Disease

Disturbances of pupillary light reflexes are classified into three groups depending on the localization of the disease process:

Those accompanying lesions of the afferent pupillary pathway

Those accompanying lesions of the midbrain (involving the pretecto-oculomotor tract)

Those accompanying lesions of the efferent pupillary pathways.

A. Lesions of the Afferent Pupillary Pathway (Table 4)

1. Failure of Retinal Function

A failure of retinal function interferes with the direct, phasic light reflex of the pupil but does not alter the consensual response. Hence the pupils are of equal size (*isocoria*). The severity of the disturbance of the light reflex corresponds to the severity of the retinal dysfunction. When retinal function is recovered, the pupillary light reflex is also restored.[14,56] With progression to complete blindness, *amaurotic pupillary akinesia* results.

TABLE 4. Pupillary Disturbances Accompanying Lesions of the Afferent Pathway

Retinal lesions	Partial interruption of conduction
Optic nerve lesions	(Pupillary light reflex diminished according to the degree of functional loss)
	Complete interruption of conduction (Amaurotic pupillary akinesia)
Optic chiasm lesions	Pupillary hemiakinesia
Optic tract lesions	Pupillary hemiakinesia

2. Lesions of the Optic Nerve

The disturbance of the pupillary light reflex corresponds to the degree of the conduction disturbance resulting from the optic nerve lesion.[96,170] As in retinal disease, the disturbance affects only the direct light reflex; a consensual reflex can still be elicited. With a complete interruption of nerve conduction, like that caused by transection, the pupil will be fixed (amaurotic pupillary akinesia). All optic nerve diseases do not affect the light reflex to an equal degree. Thus, whereas the pupil remains normal in early papilledema, it will show significant abnormalities in optic neuritis. In optic nerve diseases of vascular origin, the disturbance is relatively mild initially but will progress rapidly when the optic nerve starts to atrophy. The reason for the different pupillary effects of different optic nerve diseases relates to the structural changes occurring in the nerve itself. In the early stage of papilledema, for example, the optic disc is merely swollen by transudation, and there is no structural alteration or primary axon damage. The other opticopathies, by contrast, are associated with various optic nerve lesions in which some degree of primary axon damage has occurred.[208] There may be necrotic liquefaction of the glia and nerve fibers (ischemic opticopathy); inflammation of the nerve fibers including the medullary sheaths, axons, and glia (retrobulbar neuritis and papillitis); or loss of parenchyma with gliosis (optic atrophy).[30,87,129–132,288] The differences in the pathogenesis of the opticopathies lead to different conduction disturbances. This raises the possibility of utilizing the pupillary light reflexes as an aid to differential diagnosis. Once optic atrophy has commenced, the pupillary disturbance depends entirely on the extent and localization of the atrophy.

3. Lesions of the Optic Chiasm and Optic Tract

With lesions involving the optic chiasm and optic tract, routine examination generally will disclose no difference in the pupillary responses of both eyes. Rarely, however, a relative disturbance will be seen in the pupillary reflexes on the side opposite the tract lesion.[41] Behr reported on cases of this type as early as 1924. This phenomenon has been attributed to the greater effect of the nasal retina on pupillomotor function[252] or to a stronger representation of the nasal retina in the ipsilateral pupillomotor nucleus.[285]

An *homonymous hemianopia* caused by optic chiasm and optic tract lesions can be diagnosed pupillographically by circumscribed stimulation of the retina with small light spots to demonstrate a differential response: *pupillary hemiakinesia* (see Chapter 2, Section II).

4. Lesions of the Upper Visual Pathway

The classic notion that lesions above the lateral geniculate body do not affect the pupillary light reflexes[283] is no longer tenable. Patients with injuries of the visual cortex,[72,124–127] occipital brain injuries,[154] and infarctions of the posterior cerebral artery accompanied by CT-confirmed occipital lesions[19,226] have shown definite abnormalities of pupillomotor sensitivity in areas of visual field loss. Even circumscribed occipital infarctions with homonymous paracentral

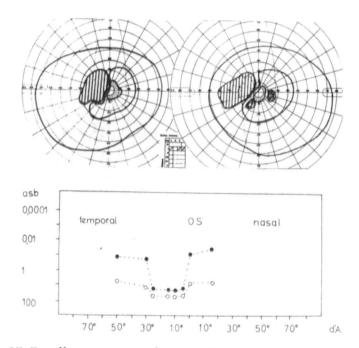

Fig. 25. Pupilloperimetry in lesions of the upper visual pathway. Pupillomotor sensitivity is diminished in the area of homonymous paracentral scotomas associated with a circumscribed occipital infarction. (After Reuther et al.[227])

scotomas lead to a considerable reduction of pupillomotor sensitivity in the affected area of the visual field (Fig. 25).

Finally, a uniform increase in the threshold for residual light perception ("blindsight")[291] and for pupillomotor function has been documented in a series of patients with "cortical amaurosis" secondary to isolated infarctions in the upper visual pathway[20] (Fig. 26).

It remains unclear whether and to what degree the pupillary light reflexes are disturbed in functional amblyopia. It is clear, however, that the severity of a pupillary defect, measurable or otherwise, does not correlate with the severity of the visual disturbance.[118,148,219]

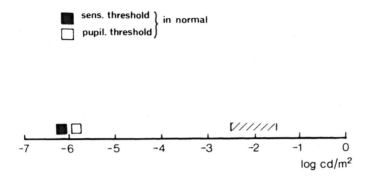

Fig. 26. Sensory and pupillomotor threshold in cortical blindness (*hatched area*). Dark adaptation. Large-field stimuli of 60°. (After Alexandridis et al. 20)

B. Examination and Differential Diagnosis of Afferent Pupillary Disturbances

If a disturbance of the afferent pupillary pathway is presumed to exist on one side, it is necessary to compare the phasic pupillary light reflexes in both eyes. When conduction is disturbed in the afferent pathway, both pupils will be equal in size (*isocoria*).

1. The Marcus Gunn Phenomenon

A complete or pronounced afferent conduction disturbance is signified by the *Marcus Gunn phenomenon*.[152] The test is performed in a brightly lit room and involves the alternate placement of a hand over each eye (Fig. 27). When the uninvolved eye is covered, there will be an immediate dilation of both pupils, since the involved eye is sending a diminished flow of impulses into the pupillomotor control circuit. When the involved eye is covered, both pupils will constrict. The Marcus Gunn phenomenon is very conspicuous in the presence of a significant, unilateral central scotoma, because, in the light-adapted eye, the key pupillomotor impulses arise from the central portions of the visual field. The

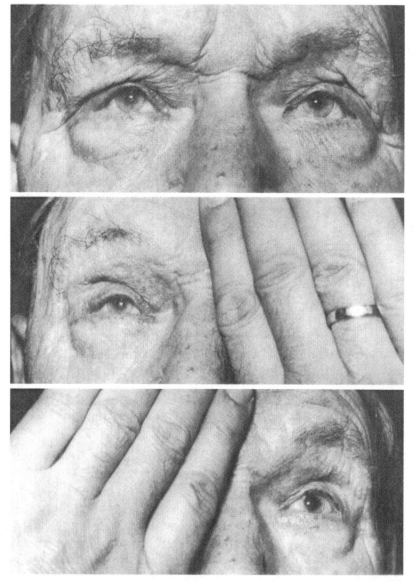

Fig. 27. Testing for the Marcus Gunn phenomenon. When the uninvolved eye is covered, both pupils dilate briskly. **Right:** Cataract with intact afferent arc. **Left:** Optic atrophy.

extreme case of the Marcus Gunn phenomenon is *amaurotic pupillary akinesia.* Since the retinal changes that produce a large, central scotoma are easily recognized, testing for the Marcus Gunn phenomenon is indicated only if optic nerve disease is suspected. Here, too, a conspicuous Marcus Gunn sign will be elicited.

2. Swinging Flashlight Test

The *swinging flashlight test*[161] is even more sensitive than the Marcus Gunn phenomenon for demonstrating very early-stage afferent pupillary defects. In this test the uninvolved eye is first illuminated eccentrically with a penlight for about 5 s, whereupon the light is swung over to the other eye. Illumination of the normal eye will cause both pupils to constrict. When the light is moved to the involved eye, both pupils will immediately dilate slightly. Returning the light to the unaffected eye will cause both pupils to constrict again, and so on (Fig. 28). This simple test is highly recommended in the office setting whenever retrobulbar neuritis is suspected. It is important that the patient not gaze at the light source so that accommodation effects are avoided. Illuminating the eye from well outside the line of vision is also useful because it produces a weak but uniform illumination of the retinal center with scattered light, while still enabling the examiner to observe the pupil clearly. In contrast to the Marcus Gunn phenomenon, this test should always be done in a dimly lit room. The swinging flashlight test is useful in differentiating papilledema from papillitis in cases where functional descriptions by the patient are inadequate for differential diagnosis. Above all, one can exclude or confirm a retrobulbar neuritis in patients who report a central scotoma but have an otherwise normal fundus.

3. Testing Pupil Cycle Time

The *pupil cycle time* is determined by measuring the duration of pupillary oscillations while directing a narrow beam

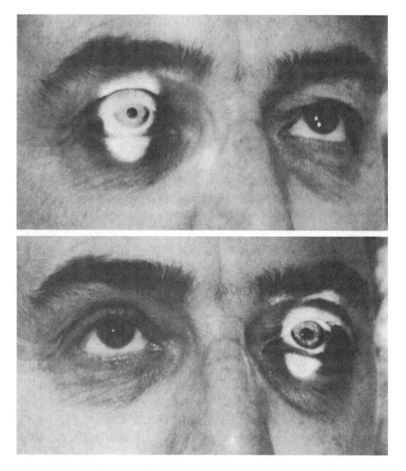

Fig. 28. The swinging flashlight test. Dilation occurs when the light is moved to the eye with poorer vision.

of light (e.g., from a slit lamp) onto the pupillary margin. A stopwatch is used to measure the duration of 100 oscillations, and the average is computed. The pupil cycle time is prolonged in the presence of optic nerve lesions.[123,191,281] It is reported that following prolonged illumination of the eye in optic neuritis, the pupillary oscillations gradually become smaller and finally cease altogether.

There are other reports that contradict these findings.[274]

Prolonged pupil cycle times have also been observed in familial dysautonomia.[103]

The pupil cycle time is prolonged by barbiturates and benzodiazepine.[238]

4. Testing the Latent Period of the Pupillary Light Reflexes

Mild functional disturbances can be objectified by testing the latent period of the pupillary light reflexes. This is done by measuring the interval between the presentation of a light stimulus and the onset of pupillary constriction.[12,29,96,170,202,265] It appears that inflammatory processes in particular, such as retrobulbar neuritis, slow the conduction velocity in the optic nerve (Fig. 29). Even after the inflammation has cleared and the visual disturbance has passed, the latent period of the light reflexes remains altered, as in the case of VEPs[16,93] The latent period of the light reflex is recorded by means of pupillography, i.e., a record of the pupillary state over time (see Chapter 2).

C. Lesions of the Midbrain (Involving the Pretecto-Oculomotor Tract)

1. Tumors

Pinealomas as well as astrocytomas and meningiomas of the quadrigeminal area lead to bilateral mydriasis with loss of the pupillary light reflexes.[237] Accommodation-convergence synkinesis is preserved. Since the pupils are large, their contraction to near vision is easily recognized. The cause is an interruption of the neurons between the pretectal nucleus and Edinger-Westphal nuclei. Dilated pupils that are unresponsive to light may be the first sign of a pineal tumor, for example, culminating in the development of a complete Parinaud syndrome in which pupillary abnormalities are accompanied by vertical gaze palsy, weakness of accommo-

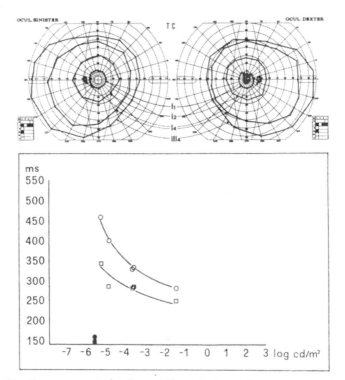

Fig. 29. Latent period of pupillary light reflexes in retrobulbar neuritis. **Top:** Relative central scotoma on the right side. **Bottom:** Latent period of the involved (O) and uninvolved eye (□) as a function of stimulus luminance. The symbols on the *abscissa* indicate the sensory thresholds of both eyes. (After Alexandridis et al.[12])

dation, and convergence-retraction nystagmus during upward gaze.

2. Tabes, Argyll Robertson Pupil

The Argyll Robertson pupil is most commonly associated with neurosyphilis, although diabetes, multiple sclerosis, encephalitis, and neoplasms may also be causative.[40] The

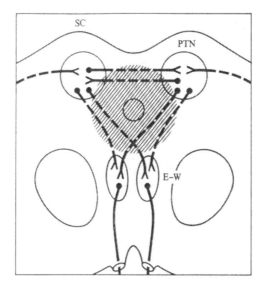

Fig. 30. Probable site of the midbrain lesion *(shaded)* in Argyll Robertson pupil. SC, Superior colliculus; PTN, pretectal nucleus; E-W, Edinger-Westphal nuclei.

lesion is probably located in the region of the Sylvian aqueduct (Fig. 30), where it interrupts the pretectal light-reflex fibers and supranuclear inhibitory fibers of the Edinger-Westphal nucleus.[279] The pupil is spastically contracted and irregular (Fig. 31). The *spastic miotic pupil* can be explained only by an interruption of supranuclear inhibition. The cortical fibers for accommodation are not affected, because they pass to the oculomotor nucleus via the superior colliculus. Accommodation-convergence synkinesis remains intact, therefore (Table 5).

A *spastic miotic pupil* may also be seen in other conditions such as arteriosclerosis, degenerative brain diseases, alcoholism, and myotonic dystrophy.[268,279] In contrast to the Argyll Robertson pupil, the pupils do not constrict with convergence, indicating that the site of the lesion is elsewhere.

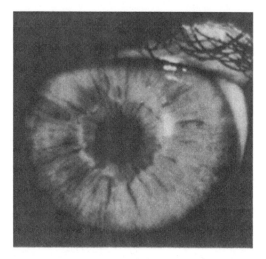

Fig. 31. Spastic miotic pupil in tabes (Argyll Robertson pupil).

D. Lesions of the Efferent Pupillary Pathways

The hallmark of efferent pupillary defects is *anisocoria* (Table 6). Not every case of anisocoria has pathologic significance, however (see Chapter 1, Section II).

TABLE 5. Pupillary Disturbances Accompanying Lesions of the Pretecto-Oculomotor Tract

Quadrigeminal tumors
Pinealomas
	{ Moderate to marked
	  mydriasis, usually
	  unilateral
		Light reflexes
		  disturbed

Neurosyphilis
(Argyll Robertson pupil)
	{ Miosis, usually
	  bilateral
		Accommodation-
		  convergence
		  synkinesis
		  intact

TABLE 6. Isocoria–Anisocoria

Isocoria	Afferent conduction disturbances	
Anisocoria	Midbrain lesions (pretecto-oculomotor tract)	
	Efferent conduction disturbances	Parasympathetic Sympathetic
	Pupillary muscle defect	

1. Lesions Involving the Parasympathetic Pupillary Fibers

The disturbance of pupillary reactions may be complete or partial, depending on the extent of the lesion. If all reflexes are lost, then *absolute pupillary akinesia* is said to be present. The causative lesion may be classified by location as preganglionic (1st neuron) or postganglionic (2nd neuron) (Table 7). Of course, both the pupillary light reflexes and accommodation-convergence synkinesis are impaired.

a. Preganglionic Lesions

The pupillomotor fibers are located in the posteromedial part of the oculomotor nucleus,[151,263] which accounts for their early involvement by compressive lesions.[40,237] Trans-

TABLE 7. Pupillary Disturbances Accompanying Lesions of the Efferent Pathway

Parasympathetic	1st Neuron		Partial interruption of conduction
	2nd Neuron (pupillotonia)		Complete interruption of conduction (absolute pupillary akinesia)
Sympathetic	Irritation (irritative mydriasis, rare)		
	Interruption	1st Neuron	
		2nd Neuron	Miosis-ptosis-enophthalmos
		3rd Neuron	(Horner syndrome)

tentorial herniations, subdural hematomas, and aneurysms of the posterior communicating artery lead to an early mydriasis with poor or absent pupillary reflexes.[40,217,262] An early disturbance of accommodation is also characteristic. A basal meningitis (tubercular or syphilitic) can also cause an isolated internal ophthalmoplegia. This paralysis is extremely rare with posterior communicating arterial aneurysms, however.[213] Generally speaking, a disturbance of the pupillary light reflex caused by a lesion of the 1st neuron will be accompanied by other disturbances in the area supplied by the oculomotor nerve. Besides transtentorial hernias, aneurysms, and subdural hematomas, these disturbances may result from infections, neoplasms, trauma, toxic effects, or other causes. With transtentorial herniations, the pupillary disturbance will sometimes be confined initially to the contralateral eye. As the hernia enlarges, the disturbance will then spread to involve the ipsilateral pupil.[192] With intracranial vascular lesions (hypertensive cerebral hemorrhage, epidural hemorrhage, cerebral infarction, etc.), an irregularity of the ipsilateral pupil may be the only sign in the early stage. Only as the patient's condition deteriorates will the complete picture of the *fixed mydriatic pupil* develop.[95] Ischemic lesions of the oculomotor nerve, like those occurring in diabetes, rarely affect the pupillomotor fibers. With lesions of the cavernous sinus, the pupil may be medium-size or even small due to concurrent sympathetic involvement, despite a profound disturbance of pupillary light reflexes.

i. Pupillary Disturbances Following Head Injuries. Ten percent of all craniocerebral injuries are associated with pupillary changes.[109] In about 50 percent of trauma patients with closed head injuries who develop hematoma-like symptoms in the absence of bleeding, a careful differentiation of pupillary signs is of substantial value.[218] In all cases the pupils should be evaluated in relation to other findings such as respiration, circulation, blood pressure and level of consciousness.[196] With direct trauma to the oculomotor nerve (ranging from contusion to transection), the pupillary disturbance is immediate and ipsilateral. Indirect oculomotor nerve damage caused by compression from transtentorial herniations develops over a period of hours or days.[262] This type of pupillary change is very common in patients with subdural and epidural hematoma and usually indicates the side of the compression.[190,191,196]

The statistical frequency of direct oculomotor nerve trauma is between 20 and 30 percent.[65,193]

Coma with a fixed pupil is an ominous sign. The prognosis is particularly grave when both pupils are dilated and unresponsive to light, in which case the mortality exceeds 85 percent. With bilateral pupillary rigidity of more than 30 minutes' duration, death is extremely likely.[218]

Very rarely, a bilateral miosis may be observed following a head injury. This is usually caused by direct trauma to the brainstem or secondary brainstem compression, a condition known as *midbrain syndrome.* The earliest manifestation of midbrain syndrome is a miosis with a very sluggish pupillary light response, presumably due to a loss of supranuclear inhibition. When fully developed, the syndrome culminates in a bilateral, fixed mydriasis. Unilateral miosis in association with ptosis and/or enophthalmos should raise the suspicion of a cervical vertebral or plexus injury (Horner Syndrome).

b. Postganglionic Lesions

i. Pupillotonia. Lesions in the postganglionic region produce the familiar picture of *pupillotonia* (tonic pupil). Females are affected more frequently than males. In about two-thirds of cases the pupillotonia is unilateral.[156,243] In ordinary daylight the tonic pupil appears larger than the contralateral, normal pupil. The pupil may show no light reflexes at all, or it may show a slow or delayed constriction to prolonged illumination, with a vermicular movement of a portion of the sphincter. This vermicular movement, which distorts the pupillary shape, is not pathognomonic, however; it may also be seen following a contusion of the globe. The convergence reaction of the tonic pupil is exaggerated in magnitude,[156] but it, too, is slow and delayed. Redilation of the pupil following far-point fixation occurs even more slowly and usually is delayed. Pupillotonia is caused by a lesion of the peripheral parasympathetic neuron. Evidently there is some degree of damage to the ciliary ganglion,[128,135,230] as is indicated by the supersensitivity of the tonic pupil to topical cholinergic stimulation. The syndrome is referred to as *acute ciliary ganglionitis*. An internal ophthalmoplegia may develop following infections, chronic tonsillitis, sinusitis, or tooth extractions. Pupillotonia has also been observed following dental anesthesia.[209] With passage of time the accommodation paresis tends to resolve in these patients, whereas the pupillary abnormality may persist. This is because 90% of the nerve fibers arising from the ciliary ganglion supply the ciliary body, but only 3% supply the sphincter pupillae.[135,230] Viral infections and syphilis have also been described as causes of ganglionitis.[135] When pupillotonia is confirmed, therefore, it is recommended that serologic tests be ordered to exclude syphilis. The pupillotonia that results from ciliary ganglionitis or injury to the ciliary ganglion cannot be distinguished from an incidentally discovered pupillotonia of unknown etiology.

ii. Adie Syndrome. Adie syndrome is the term applied to idiopathic pupillotonia (tonic pupil associated with ciliary ganglionitis of unknown cause) accompanied by an impairment of deep tendon reflexes. In rare cases segmental hypohidrosis (Ross syndrome) has been described in addition to the tonic pupil and decreased tendon reflexes.[133,181,215,234] Contrary to classic beliefs, the reflex abnormalities are not confined to the knee and ankle, but may affect the upper extremity as well.[267] Idiopathic pupillotonia with normal tendon reflexes is not considered to be a separate entity. In the American literature, therefore, all cases of idiopathic pupillotonia are grouped under the heading of Adie syndrome, regardless of whether or not tendon reflexes are impaired. Loewenfeld et al.[168] state that in 11% of patients, unilateral pupillotonia is only one symptom of a more complex disease process. With bilateral pupillotonia, the incidence is around 60%. Bilateral pupillotonia with impaired accommodation is seen frequently in Charcot-Marie-Tooth disease [60,149] and may also occur in association with giant-cell arteritis.[58,79]

iii. Abnormalities of the Sphincter Pupillae. Congenital abnormalities of the sphincter are very rare. They lead to anisocoria and varying degrees of pupillary light reflex impairment. Contusions of the eyeball and exposure to pupil-active drugs must always be excluded as causes of unilateral mydriasis with loss of pupillary reflexes.

Relative pupillary disturbances are observed in myasthenia gravis due to hyposensitivity of the cholinergic receptors.[287]

2. Lesions of the Sympathetic Nervous System

a. Interruption of the Sympathetic Pathway, Horner Syndrome

An interruption of sympathetic innervation occurring in the setting of Horner syndrome leads to ipsilateral paralytic miosis. The direct and consensual light reflexes are unaffected, and the pupil constricts normally to near vision. Horner syndrome is easily recognized from the characteristic triad of miosis, mild ptosis, and enophthalmos (Fig. 32). The narrowing of the palpebral fissure and ptosis result from a paresis of Müller's smooth orbital muscle. Both the dilator pupillae and the Müller muscle are supplied by the same cervical sympathetic trunk (Fig. 3). Other signs of lost sympathetic innervation are: vasodilation of the conjunctiva and ipsilateral facial half, hypohidrosis, and, in younger individuals, heterochromia iridis.

Hypohidrosis of the face and neck signifies a cervical sympathetic lesion. If sweat secretion on the arm is also af-

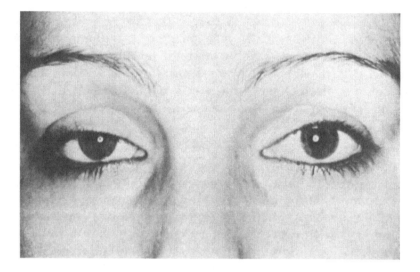

Fig. 32. Horner syndrome. Miosis, ptosis, enophthalmos.

fected, a lesion of the stellate ganglion is indicated. If sweat secretion is not disturbed in a postganglionic Horner syndrome, the lesion must be located above the carotid bifurcation and thus in the area of the internal carotid artery, cavernous sinus, or orbital floor.

Numerous pathologic processes of various types, including neoplasms, infections, and trauma occurring in any of the three neuronal regions may produce the syndrome. Herpes zoster or inflammations involving the cavernous sinus may also be causative.[141,145] If the lesion is central or preganglionic in location, i.e., located in the area of the 1st and 2nd neuron of the sympathetic pathway, then the likelihood of a malignancy is high. Approximately half of preganglionic lesions are malignant tumors.[106,110,119] A frequent cause of Horner syndrome in the area of the 1st neuron is vertebrobasilar insufficiency in a setting of Wallenberg syndrome (dorsolateral oblongata syndrome). Severe cervical spondylosis and vehicular "whiplash" injuries are typical mechanisms that can cause Horner syndrome through lesions of the 1st neuron. Apical pulmonary carcinoma (Pancoast syndrome) and mediastinal tumors can interrupt the sympathetic pathway in the region of the 2nd neuron and produce a Horner syndrome.

With a postganglionic lesion, it is likely that the disease process is vascular in nature. Frequently these patients suffer histamine or "cluster" headaches[92] or experience attacks of unilateral headache in the setting of Raeder's paratrigeminal syndrome.[74,119]

Raeder's paratrigeminal syndrome, which is characterized by episodes of severe unilateral headache distributed in the 1st or 2nd division of the trigeminal nerve associated with the signs of Horner syndrome, predominantly affects middle-aged and elderly men. The pain attacks occur at night or early in the morning, accompanied by nausea and vomiting. Usually the attacks disappear spontaneously in a few weeks or months, but the Horner syndrome tends to persist. If Raeder syndrome is accompanied by disturbances in the region of the 3rd, 4th, 5th, or 6th nerve, it is necessary that a malignancy be excluded.[120]

b. Sympathetic Irritation

In very rare cases an irritative lesion of the sympathetic pathway will produce a "reverse" Horner syndrome with widening of the palpebral fissure and mydriasis.[40,279] An apical pneumonitis is usually present. Pupillary light reflexes are not affected.

E. Pharmacodynamic Tests for the Differential Diagnosis of Efferent Pupillary Disturbances

The patient with anisocoria will usually have a lesion of the efferent pupillomotor pathway (Table 7). The first step in evaluating such a patient in the office setting is to darken the room and see whether the pupillary inequality increases (with the large pupil dilating further) or decreases (with the small pupil becoming larger). The former signifies involvement of the smaller pupil, and the latter involvement of the larger pupil.

The next step is to test the pupillary light reflexes. The slit lamp is excellent for this purpose in the office setting. Either both pupils will react promptly, or one pupil will react sluggishly or not at all. If one of the pupils shows an abnormal light reaction, the accommodation-convergence reflex of that pupil should be tested. If the pupil does not show marked constriction on accommodation, the synkinesis is pathologic (Fig. 33).

1. Larger Pupil is Abnormal

Let us assume that the larger pupil reacts slowly or not at all to light and to near vision. In this case a disturbance of the parasympathetic nervous system or of the iris musculature may be presumed. The next step is to localize the lesion. This is done by means of a pharmacodynamic test:

a. Pilocarpine Test

Pilocarpine in 0.2% solution is instilled into both eyes. Normally this concentration will not produce a visible alteration of pupil size. Marked constriction of the pupil on the affected side in response to pilocarpine signifies a denervation hypersensitivity of the muscle receptor. The lesion in such cases is postganglionic, and pupillotonia may be diagnosed. If the pupil is unresponsive to pilocarpine, the lesion must be located either in the 1st neuron of the oculomotor nerve or in the iris musculature. This question is resolved by reinstilling pilocarpine into each eye, this time in 1% solution. If now the pupil on the affected side constricts promptly, like its fellow, the lesion must involve the 1st neuron of the oculomotor nerve. If the pupil shows little or no change relative to its fellow, a lesion of the iris muscle is signified (cf. Fig. 33). It will then be necessary to exclude

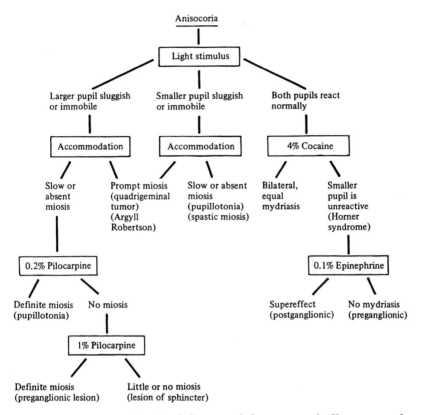

Fig. 33. Flow chart for the differential diagnosis of efferent pupillary defects.

trauma or contamination with mydriatics. Congenital anomalies of the iris muscles are very rare.

b. Cocaine-Pilocarpine Test

If pupillotonia is suspected in the presence of a small pupil, the cocaine-pilocarpine test is diagnostic. It is performed by first instilling 2% cocaine into both eyes, followed 30 min later by 0.5% pilocarpine (or 0.75% carbachol) (Fig. 34). Mydriasis following cocaine would preclude a diagnosis of reflex pupillary paralysis. The main value of the test, how-

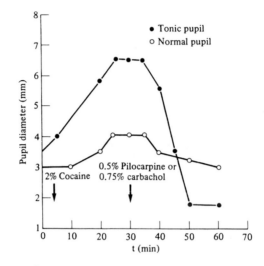

Fig. 34. The cocaine-pilocarpine test for pupillotonia.

ever, is its superior capacity to demonstrate supersensitivity to pilocarpine. Testing to exclude a lesion of the 1st neuron (with 1% pilocarpine), if required, should be deferred for at least a day.

c. Mecholyl Test

The mecholyl test is particularly valuable when bilateral pupillotonia is suspected.[3,243] The diagnosis is confirmed by a strong miosis after the instillation of a 2.5% solution. In the absence of pupillotonia, no reaction will occur. Mecholyl, unfortunately, is no longer produced commercially.

If the large pupil does not respond to light yet constricts well on accommodation, then a *light-reflex pupillary akinesia* is present. This condition is usually bilateral and signifies a lesion of the midbrain (quadrigeminal tumor). In other cases it may represent an early-stage Argyll Robertson pupil.

2. Smaller Pupil is Abnormal

Let us now assume that the smaller pupil reacts poorly to light but shows a brisk accommodation-convergence synkinesis. This is the classic picture of the Argyll Robertson pupil in tabes (cf. Fig. 33).

If the small pupil does not react to accommodation, one must again entertain a diagnosis of pupillotonia and carry out the appropriate pharmacodynamic test.

3. Both Pupils React Normally

If both pupils react briskly to light, two possibilities exist: simple anisocoria without pathologic significance, or Horner syndrome. In any case it is necessary first to establish whether or not the anisocoria is pathologic.

a. Cocaine Test

Cocaine is instilled into each eye in 4% solution. The cocaine enhances the effect of endogenous norepinephrine by blocking its reabsorption at nerve terminals. Either both pupils will respond with mydriasis, or the small pupil will show little or no response.[242] In the first case the anisocoria is considered to have no pathologic significance; in the second case, a Horner syndrome is indicated (Fig. 35; see also Fig. 33). The next step would be to localize the lesion to a particular site in the sympathetic pathway. This will aid greatly in clarifying the etiology of the disorder. If the lesion involves the 3rd neuron, and thus the neuron in closest proximity to the pupil, then hypersensitivity to epinephrine will be particularly evident.

b. Epinephrine Test

A 0.1% epinephrine solution is sufficient to cause pronounced mydriasis on the side with the small pupil, but it will not affect the normal pupil. If the epinephrine solution

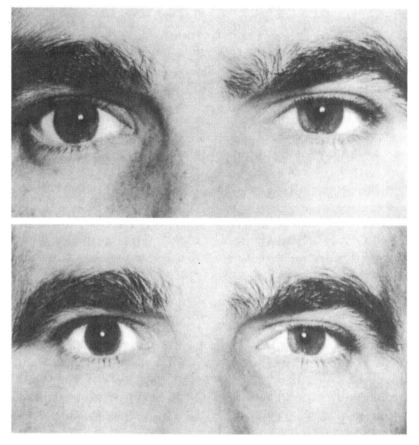

Fig. 35. The cocaine test in Horner syndrome. Note absence of mydriasis on the involved side (**bottom**).

produces no effect, the lesion must be preganglionic, i.e., either central or involving the 2nd neuron (Table 8).

c. Hydroxyamphetamine Test

An alternative to epinephrine is hydroxyamphetamine instilled in 1% solution. With a preganglionic lesion, both pupils will dilate equally following hydroxyamphetamine. With a postganglionic lesion, the pupil on the side with the sympathetic nerve lesion will remain small.[266]

TABLE 8. Pharmacodynamics of Horner Syndrome

| | Intact sympathetic pathway | Lesion of Sympathetic Pathway | | |
| | | Preganglionic | | Post-ganglionic 3rd neuron |
		1st Neuron	2nd Neuron	
Cocaine 4%	Mydriasis	Little effect	No effect	No effect
Epinephrine 0.1%	Little or no effect	No effect	Very little or no effect	Mydriasis
Hydroxyam-phetamine 1%	Mydriasis	Mydriasis	Mydriasis	No effect

It should be pointed out that none of the foregoing pharmacologic effects is 100% reliable as a localizing sign in Horner syndrome.[186]

F. Periodic Pupillary Disturbances

1. Hippus

Besides physiologic pupillary unrest, whose oscillations are slow and of small magnitude, a similar but more pronounced phenomenon may be observed in various neurologic disorders as well as in normal individuals: sudden, rhythmic changes in pupil size, sometimes amounting to 2–3 mm. This state of heightened pupillary unrest is called *hippus*. It is unaffected by light, convergence, or psychosensory stimuli. Hippus has been seen in association with multiple sclerosis, syphilis of the brain, progressive paralysis, acute meningitis, epilepsy, myasthenia gravis, and quadrigeminal tumors.[44,89,279] According to Bing,[43] hippus is based on a subcortical extrapyramidal hyperkinesia, which may be present in asymptomatic individuals. Hippus sometimes occurs as a toxic drug effect (see Section III).

2. Springing Pupil

Another type of periodic pupillary disturbance is the *springing pupil,* in which the pupils become markedly dilated in alternating fashion, showing little or no light reaction during the dilatory phase. The transient mydriasis may be confined to one side. This is a very rare phenomenon which occurs in the setting of purely functional disease states, especially psychoneurotic ones.[66] Neurosyphilis and poisonings may also have causal significance.[89,279] The pathogenesis of the phenomenon is unknown. Distortions of pupil shape lasting for several minutes have also been reported. This disturbance is based on a transitory sympathetic irritation of unknown cause. Horner syndrome, pupillotonia, or migraine is present in most patients.[269]

G. Paradoxical Pupillary Reactions

A paradoxical pupillary reaction is one in which the pupil dilates on exposure to light and constricts in the dark. It is an extremely rare phenomenon. Many such cases are reported in the older literature, but the majority are probably the result of faulty observation.[44] Central nervous system causes, including syphilis, have been cited most frequently as etiologic factors.[38,39,63,169,205,279] The pathogenesis remains unclear. Peripheral lesions have also been implicated as causing unilateral paradoxical light reactions.[99,110,207] Cases of this type are not uncommon[80,99,113,207,210] and usually are based on an aberrant regeneration of oculomotor nerves supplying the external ocular muscles. The pupil on the affected side is generally unreactive to light and shows only slight miosis on near vision (pseudo-Argyll Robertson syndrome). The defect occurs when the sphincter pupillae gains innervation from oculomotor fibers that normally supply the external ocular muscles. As a result, ocular movements in the direction of action of the involved muscle cause certain sectors of the sphincter to contract.

Transient miosis immediately after dark in night blindness[36] and in achromatopsia[97] has also been reported.

H. Pupillary Disturbance in Epilepsy

The *fixed mydriatic pupil* is a condition where the dilator pupillae is in a state of sustained contraction due to supranuclear inhibition of the Edinger-Westphal nucleus. All pupillary light reflexes are absent or profoundly impaired. The fixed mydriatic pupil is observed during grand mal seizures as well as petit mal episodes.[143] Usually the disturbance is , bilateral, although a unilateral dilation has been described.[211]

III. Pupillary Disturbances Due to Poisonings

Pupillary disturbances due to toxic effects usually affect both eyes equally. Anisocoria is rare. The most common disturbance is mydriasis, accompanied by a loss or reduction of the phasic light reflex and an impairment of accommodation (Table 9). When an anticholinergic effect occurs, both the tonic and phasic light reflexes will be disturbed to an equal degree. With an adrenergic effect, the tonic light reflex will be disturbed to a relatively greater degree. With toxic damage to the afferent pupillary pathway (e.g., the optic nerve or retina), all the light reflexes will be impaired to some degree, with amaurotic pupillary paralysis representing the extreme case.

Miosis is a less frequent consequence of poisonings (Table 10). In accordance with initial pupil size, the phasic light reflex will be reduced or, as in the spastic tonic pupil, absent.

A. Poisonings Characterized by Mydriasis

1. Drug Side Effects

As in almost all poisonings, the pupillary disturbances from drug side effects are bilateral and equal. The most important drugs to be considered are those that produce mydriasis as a side effect.

TABLE 9. Poisonings Characterized by Mydriasis

Drug side effects:	Antispasmodics, antiparkinson drugs, antidepressants, tranquilizers, CNS stimulants
Botulism	
Plant poisonings:	Belladona, *Vaccinium uliginosum*, horse chestnut, arum, bitter-sweet, nightshade, snakeweed, *Euphorbia*
Mushroom poisonings	
Chemical substances:	Carbon monoxide, DDT, tetramethyl butanediamide
Lead poisoning	
Snakebite	

Sometimes the same drug can produce both mydriasis and miosis as a side effect. Many drugs that act on the central nervous system can cause pupillary dilation or constriction, depending on the dosage. Hippus is a possible but uncommon drug side effect. The pharmaceutical industry states that glaucoma is a contraindication to all such products. However, it is necessary to make a distinction between patients already diagnosed as having glaucoma and those who are predisposed to glaucoma attack.

Most patients with recognized glaucoma are already being treated medically with miotic or beta-blocking drugs, or possibly their condition has beens surgically cured. When the intraocular pressure is well controlled, the systemic use of anticholinergic drugs poses no significant risk, especially

TABLE 10. Poisonings Characterized by Miosis

Drug side effects	Analgesics, narcotics, antihypertensives, antimyasthenics
Plant poisonings:	*Paris quadrifolia*, marihuana smoke
Mushroom poisonings	
Agricultural pesticides:	Parathion (E-605), Meta-Systox
Chemical weapons:	Sarin, tabun
Scorpion venom	

in patients who are taking miotics. Even less danger is posed by the systemic use of adrenergic drugs, provided the pupil is adequately constricted by miotics. In cases where glaucoma has been successfully managed by surgery, mydriasis can have no adverse consequences. It is true that many patients with very narrow anterior chamber angles still experience glaucoma attacks despite the use of miotics. However, the majority of these patients are those who are predisposed to glaucoma by their narrow chamber angles but have previously been unaware of that condition.

It would be impractical to require that every patient undergo a preliminary ophthalmologic examination to exclude predisposition to glaucoma attack before such drugs are prescribed. However, a preliminary examination might be appropriate in elderly patients, who constitute a relatively high-risk group, and this would be particularly advised in cases where long-term treatment with an anticholinergic agent (e.g., antiparkinson drugs) is proposed.

a. Antispasmodics

Mydriasis, a weak or absent light reflex, and impaired accommodation may occur following the systemic use of antispasmodics for the treatment of gastrointestinal disorders. Given their frequent and widespread usage, these drugs (especially the belladona alkaloids) are notorious for their capacity to precipitate glaucoma in eyes having narrow anterior chamber angles.[275] The most important of these drugs are: atropine, amprotropine, glycopyrrolate, isopropamide, methixene,[98,115,116,179,272] methantheline,[199] diphemanil, metcaraphen, ambutonium bromide, oxyphenonium, oxyphencyclimine, orphenadrine, and others.[50,98,116,137]

b. Antiparkinson Drugs

The antiparkinson drugs merit special attention, for they are used predominantly in elderly patients who are at increased risk for glaucoma. The drugs caramiphen, cycrimine, ethy-

benzatropine, profenamine, biperiden, benztropine, chlor-
phenoxamine, procyclidine, and trihexyphenidyl can produce an atropine-like anticholinergic side effect resulting in mydriasis with loss of the phasic pupillary reflex.[115,116,158,179,272,279]

It is reported that levo-3,4-dihydroxyphenylalanine (L-
DOPA) also used in the treatment of parkinsonism, causes
both mydriasis and a widening of the palpebral fissure as
part of its sympathomimetic effect.[111,286] By accentuating a
preexisting, subclinical lateral discrepancy of sympathetic
innervation, the drug can cause Horner-type symptoms to
appear.[282] Accommodation is unaffected. Miosis during L-
DOPA therapy has also been described.[255]

c. Antidepressants

The danger of mydriasis following the use of tricyclic anti-
depressants such as amitriptyline, nortriptyline, and pro-
triptyline is well documented.[82,116,271,272] The antidepressant
imipramine has anticholinergic activity even in ordinary
doses.[82,116]

d. Tranquilizers

An anticholinergic effect is attributed to pecazine, a
phenothiazine-derivative tranquilizer. It leads to mydriasis
with a disturbance of the phasic pupillary light reflex and
impaired accommodation.[116] Overdosage of meprobamate
can also cause mydriasis.[82,116,272]

e. Central Nervous System Stimulants

Amphetamine, a synthetic central nervous system stimulant
with adrenergic properties, can cause mydriasis when administered in large doses.[237] At the same time, it has been
observed that patients with Argyll Robertson syndrome re-
gain a normal pupillary light reaction following treatment
with amphetamine.[279] Dexamphetamine can also dilate the

pupils and disturb pupillary reflexes when given in excessive dosage.[116] Mydriasis has been observed during shock therapy with pentylenetetrazol.[199]

f. Other Drugs that Cause Mydriasis

Mydriasis and a weakened phasic light reflex have been observed following the administration of emetine for the treatment of amebiasis,[98,116,279] ganglion-blocking drugs,[35,272] the appetite suppressants fenfluramine and phenmetrazine,[98,115,116] and in some instances following the use of antihistamines.[98,115,116,237] Transient pupillotonia with heightened sensitivity to cholinergic agents has been reported following quinine poisonings.[105]

Hallucinogens such as lysergic acid diethylamine (LSD) can produce a sympathetic mydriasis.[98,116]

The anticonvulsant phenytoin, when given in excessive dosage, leads to ataxia, nystagmus, convulsions, and frequently mydriasis.[212]

2. Botulism

Botulism toxin adheres to the synapses of parasympathetic nerve fibers and inhibits the synthesis of acetylcholine.[59,71] This leads to a range of morbid ophthalmic signs in which oculomotor paralysis is predominant: mydriasis with loss of light reflexes and convergence synkinesis, accommodation paralysis, strabismus, diplopia, and ptosis. The pupillary disturbances may persist for some months following the clinical resolution of other symptoms.[121] Mydriasis is not always present.[199] Abducens paralysis ranging to complete ophthalmoplegia has been reported.[199]

3. Plant Poisonings

Besides acute atropine poisoning, which is most commonly seen in children who have eaten berries from *Atropa bella-*

dona, there are a number of other plants that have toxic effects involving the pupil.

Berries from the shrub *Vaccinium uliginosum*, which are found in the marshlands of the Alpine foothills and resemble blueberries, cause impaired accommodation and mydriasis when ingested in quantities of 250–350 g.[199]

Ingestion of berries and leaves from the arum plant (*Aron maculatum*) causes mydriasis. Fatalities have been reported, especially in children.

Horse chestnuts (*Aesculus hippocastanum*) are particularly dangerous to small children because of their content of saponins. Poisonings are associated with mydriasis.[248]

Mydriasis also results from the ingestion of bittersweet (*Solanum dulcanara*) and nightshade (*Solanum negrum*), which contain the alkaloid solanin,[116] and from poisoning with snakeweed. All *Euphorbia* species contain a bitter milky juice which, when ingested, produces multiple toxic symptoms and mydriasis.

4. Mushroom Poisoning

Published reports on the pupillary effects of mushroom poisonings are contradictory. This may be the result of regional differences in the alkaloid content of certain species. *Amanita pantherina*, for example, causes no muscarine-like effects, but it contains an alkaloid that produces an atropine-like poisoning. The victim becomes manic and erethismic, the pupils dilate, and pupillary reflexes are lost.[199]

5. Chemical Poisonings

a. Carbon Monoxide

One effect of acute poisoning is mydriasis.

b. Tetramethyl Butanediamine

Workers exposed to tetramethyl butanediamine fumes have developed corneal irritation and photophobia, as well as mydriasis and accommodation disturbances.[112,251]

c. DDT (Dichlorodiphenyltrichloroethane)

The toxicology of DDT resembles that of strychnine. Severe cases are associated with extreme mydriasis. The pupils are of unequal size, and they are unreactive to light and convergence.[199]

6. Lead Poisoning

Blatt noted mydriasis and impaired reflexes in 21 of 320 patients with lead poisoning, and accommodation disturbances in two. None of these patients suffered any vision impairment.[48]

7. Snakebite

The bites of many snakes with neurotropic venom cause ptosis, impaired accommodation, and oculomotor paralysis, as well as mydriasis and disturbed pupillary light reflexes.[27,47,229] Complete ophthalmoplegia has also been described as a sequel to snakebite.[114,200,224]

B. Poisonings Characterized by Miosis

1. Drug Side Effects

a. Narcotics and Analgesics

All opiates such as codeine, cyclazocine, heroin, methadone, morphine, pentazocine, and pethidine exert a miotic action.[67] It is assumed that the miosis results from a direct effect on pupillomotor centers.[241] Opiate antagonists such as levallorphan, nalorphine, and naloxone, which are given systemically to relieve respiratory depression following general anesthesia, also cause miosis when administered alone. They cause mydriasis only if miosis has been previously induced by the administration of opiates.[98,116,187,199]

b. Antimyasthenic Drugs

The cholinesterase inhibitors physostigmine, neostigmine, pyridostygmine, and tetraethylpyrophosphate (TEPP), which are used in the treatment of myasthenia, can produce a miosis similar to that caused by topically applied cholinesterase inhibitors.[98,115,116,272]

c. Antihypertensive Drugs

Guanethidine, used systemically in the treatment of hypertension, exerts an antiadrenergic effect that leads to miosis, sometimes to the point of mild ptosis and conjunctival hyperemia like that seen in Horner syndrome.[98,116,199,231,272] Miosis may also occur following the systemic administration of phenoxybenzamine, an α-blocking drug.[98,115,116,279] Reserpine, which is used both as an antihypertensive and as a tranquilizer, can occasionally cause mild miosis.[98,116]

2. Plant Poisoning

The berries of *Paris quadrifolia* are often confused with belladona. They are relatively harmless, causing moderate gastrointestinal disturbances and miosis. The smoking of marihuana constricts the pupils through a sympathetic disturbance.[136]

3. Mushroom Poisoning

The ingestion of poisonous mushrooms such as *Amanita muscaria* produces a typical muscarine syndrome with sweating, salivation, and miosis.[116,199,284]

4. Pesticides

The most familiar and dangerous of the agricultural pesticides are parathion (E-605) and Meta-Systox. They belong to the class of alkyl phosphates and are cholinesterase inhibitors. Acute poisonings, which often have a fatal outcome, cause extreme miosis in addition to other toxic symptoms.[116,199,250]

5. Chemical Weapons

Inhalation of the nerve gases sarin and tabun has various effects including spasm of accommodation and miosis. These gases are classified chemically as alkyl phosphates.[116,199]

6. Scorpion Venom

Different scorpion venoms vary greatly in their effect. Strabismus and diplopia have been reported in severe cases. Miosis is a constant finding in highly poisonous stings.[116]

C. Hippus and Episodic Pupillary Changes Due to Poisonings

1. Drug Side Effects

Both mydriasis and miosis can occur as side effects of the same drug. Many drugs that act on the central nervous system can cause mydriasis or miosis, depending on the dosage. Hippus is a rare but definite side effect of certain drugs.

a. Sedatives and Hypnotics

The numerous barbiturate preparations and barbiturate derivatives, which are widely used as sedatives and hypnotics, vary considerably in the intensity of their side effects. At ordinary dose levels the pupil is seldom affected. Overdosage or long-term use can lead to mydriasis with weakening of the phasic pupillary light reflex. Miosis is equally common, however. Hippus has been frequently described as a side effect of barbiturates,[64,98,116,247] and anisocoria has been noted in association with barbiturate poisoning.[98]

The bromides frequently cause mydriasis when given in overdose; miosis is less common. Hippus has also been observed.[116,162] Overdosage of glutethimide has been associated with cerebellar ataxia, nystagmus, and mydriasis with a severe disturbance of the phasic light reflex.[116,147] Finally, miosis results from the central effects of a mild overdose of chloralhydrate and paraldehyde, whereas mydriasis is characteristic of a heavier overdose.[84,116,162,237,241,273]

b. Tranquilizers and Antipsychotics

Phenothiazine derivatives are the most widely prescribed agents, with chlorpromazine ranking first. These drugs cause ocular side effects including miosis and mydriasis in about 30% of patients who have been taking the medication for several years.[67,84,98,116,279] Meprobamate, a tranquilizer, can induce a coma-like state when given in excessive dosage. The pupils in this state vary greatly in their behavior, showing mydriasis or miosis, a normal phasic light reflex or an absent reflex, and possibly anisocoria.[107,116]

c. Anticonvulsants

In primidone poisoning, hippus has been observed in addition to a somnolent state of consciousness.[204]

d. Oral Contraceptives

The ocular side effects of oral contraceptives are varied and include mydriasis resulting from an afferent arc disturbance, miosis in the setting of a complete Horner syndrome, and anisocoria.[84,98,116,137,158,237]

References

1. Abelsdorf G (1900) Die Änderungen der Pupillenweite durch verschiedenfarbige Belichtung. Z Psychol Physiol Sinnesorg 22:81–95
2. Abelsdorf G (1919) Zur Frage der Existenz besonderer Pupillarfasern im Sehnerven. Klin Monatsbl Augenheilkd 62:170–175
3. Adler FH, Scheie H (1940) The site of the disturbance in tonic pupils. Trans Am Ophthalmol Soc 38:183–192
4. Aguilar M, Stiles NS (1954) Saturation of the rod mechanism of the retina at high levels of stimulation. Optica Acta 1:59–65
5. Alexandridis E (1967) Pupillographische Untersuchung der Netzhautempfindlichkeit des Taubenauges. Albrecht von Graefes Arch Klin Ophthalmol 172:139–151
6. Alexandridis E (1967) Pupillographische Untersuchung der Netzhautempfindlichkeit eines Stäbchenmonochromaten. Pflügers Arch Ges Physiol 294:67
7. Alexandridis E (1968) Bestimmung der Dunkeladaptationskurve mit Hilfe der Pupillenlichtreflexe. Ber Dtsch Ophthalmol Ges 68:274–277
8. Alexandridis E (1970) Räumliche und zeitliche Summation pupillomotorisch wirksamer Lichtreize beim Menschen. Albrecht von Graefes Arch Klin Ophthalmol 18:12–19
9. Alexandridis E (1970) Spektrale Empfindlichkeit der Pupillenlichtreflexe eines Stäbchenmonochromten. Ber Dtsch Ophthalmol Ges 70:580–583
10. Alexandridis E (1971) Pupillographie. Anwendungsmöglichkeiten als objektive Untersuchungsmethode der Netzhautsinnesfunktion. Hüthig. Heidelberg

11. Alexandridis E (1973) Lichtsinn und Pupillenreaktion. In:
    Dodt E, Schrader KE (Hrsg) Die normale und die gestörte
    Pupillenbewegung Bergmann, München
12. Alexandridis E, Argyropoulos Tr, Krastel H (1981) The latent
    period of the pupil light reflex in lesions of the optic nerve.
    Ophthalmologica 182:2 1–217
13. Alexandridis E, Baumann Ch (1967) Wirkliche und schein-
    bare Pupillenweiten des menschlichen Auges. Optica Acta
    14:311–316
14. Alexandridis E, Bischoff M (1975) Sensorische und pupillo-
    motorische Empfindlichkeit nach operativer Behandlung der
    Netzhautablösung. Mod Probl Ophthalmol 15:300–303
15. Alexandridis E, Dodt E (1967) Pupillenlichtreflexe und Pu-
    pillenweite einer Stäbchenmonochromatin. Albrecht von
    Graefes Arch Klin Ophthalmol 173:153–161
16. Alexandridis E, Gärtner RL, Krastel H, Hagenlocher H-U
    (1982) Latenz der Pupillenlichtreflexe und des VECP im
    Verlauf der retrobulbären Neuritis. Fortschr Augenheilkd
    79:356–357
17. Alexandridis E, Koeppe ER (1969) Die spektrale Emp-
    findlichkeit der für den Pupillenlichtreflex verantworthli-
    chen Photorezeptoren beim Menschen. Albrecht von
    Graefes Arch Klin Ophthalmol 177:136–151
18. Alexandridis E, Krastel H (1972) Ein tragbares Infrarot-Re-
    flex-Pupillometer. Ber Dtsch Ophthalmol Ges 71:652–654
19. Alexandridis E, Krastel H, Reuther R (1979) Pupillenreflex-
    störungen bei Läsionen der oberen Sehbahn. Albrecht von
    Graefes Arch Klin Ophthalmol 209:199–208
20. Alexandridis E, Krastel H, Reuther R (1983) In wieweit sind
    die Pupillenlichtreflexe bei der kortikalen Amaurose gestört?
    Fortschr Ophthalmol 80:79–81
21. Alexandridis E, Manner M (1977) Folgefrequenz der Pupille
    bei flimmernden Lichtreizen. Albrecht von Graefes Arch
    Klin Ophthalmol 202:175–180
22. Alexandridis E, Weddigen A (1971) Pupillenlichtreflexe bei
    Heredodegeneratio pigmentosa retinae. Albrecht von
    Graefes Arch Klin Ophthalmol 182:250–260
23. Alfonso GF (1963) Pupillometria all' infrarosso mediante
    convertitore d'immagini. Riv Otoneuro Oftalmol 38:595–604
24. Alkemade PPH (1969) Dysgenesis mesodermalis of the iris
    and the cornea. Koninklijke, Van Gorcum, Assen

25. Alpern M, Benson DJ (1953) Directional sensitivity of the pupillomotor photoreceptors. Am J Optom Physiol Opt 30:569–580

26. Alpern M, Campbell FW (1962) The spectral sensitivity of the consensual light reflex. J Physiol (Lond) 169:478–507

27. Alvaro ME (1939) Snake venom in ophthalmology. Am J Opthalmol 22:1130–1146

28. Apter JT (1956) Studies of the autonomic innervation of the iris. Am J Ophthalmol 42:122–130

29. Argyropoulos Tr, Krastel H, Alexandridis E (1980) Latenz der Pupillenlichtreflexe bei Erkrankungen des Sehnerven. Ber Dtsch Ophthalmol Ges 77:373–377

30. Arieff A (1955) Pathways of darkness and reflex pupillary dilatation. Am J Ophthalmol 40:119–120

31. Ariëns Kappers J (1973) Die zentrale Regulierung der normalen Pupillenbewegung. In: Dodt E, Schrader KE (Hrsg) Die normale und die gestörte Pupillenbewegung. Bergmann, München

32. Asano J, Finnila CA, Sever G, Stanten S, Stark L, Willis PA (1962) Pupillometry. Q Rep Electronics 66:404–412

33. Atchison D, Smith G, Efron N (1979) The effect of pupil size on visual acuity in uncorrected and corrected myopia. Am J Optom Physiol Opt 56:315–323

34. Aulhorn E (1967) Die Abhängigkeit der Sehschärfe von der Pupillenweite. Ber Dtsch Ophthalmol Ges 68:304–309

35. Barnett AJ (1952) Ocular effects of methonium compounds. Br J Ophthalmol 36:593–602

36. Baricks ME, Flynn JT, Kushner BJ (1971) Paradoxical pupillary responses in congenital stationary night blindness. In: Smith JL (ed) Neuro-ophthalmology update. Masson, New York

37. Barris RW (1936) A pupillo-constrictor area in the cerebral cortex of the cat and its relationship to the pretectal area. J Comp Neurol 63:353–368

38. Behr C (1922) Die paradoxe Lichtreaktion der Pupille. Klin Monatsbl Augenheilkd 69:189–205

39. Behr C (1924) Die Lehre von den Pupillenbewegungen. In: Graefe-Saemisch (Hrsg) Handbuch der gesamten Augenheilkunde, Bd II: Die Untersuchungsmethoden. Springer, Berlin

40. Behrens MM (1977) Failure of the light reaction. Trans Am Acad Ophthalmol Otolaryngol 83:827–831
41. Bell RA, Thompson HS (1978) Relative afferent pupillary defect in optic tract hemianopsias. Am J Ophthalmol 85:538–540
42. Bellarminoff L (1885) Anwendung der graphischen Methode bei Untersuchung der Pupillenbewegungen. Photocoreograph. Pflügers Arch Ges Physiol 37:107–122
43. Benevento LA, Rezah M, Santos-Andersen R (1977) An autoradiographic study of the projections of the pretectum in the rhesus monkey (Macaca mulatta): evidence for sensorimotor links to the thalamus and oculomotor nuclei. Brain Res 127:197–218
44. Bing R, Franceschetti A (1931) Die Pupille. In: Schieck E, Brückner A (Hrsg) Kurzes Handbuch der Ophthalmologie, Bd VI. Springer, Berlin
45. Birmingham AT, Szolcsanyi J (1965) Competitive blockade of adrenergic α-receptors and histamine receptors by thymoxamine. J Pharm Pharmacol 17:449–458
46. Birren JE, Casperson RC, Botwinick J (1950) Age changes in pupil size. J Gerontol 5:216–225
47. Blatt N (1922) Zur Kasuistik der Augenveränderungen bei Vergiftung durch Schlanbenbiß. Z Augenheilkd 49:280–282
48. Blatt N (1931) Akkommodationslähmungen und Pupillenstörungen nach Bleivergiftung. Klin Monatsbl Augenheilkd 86:482–491
49. Bleichert A, Wagner R (1957) Versuche zur Erfassung des Pupillenspiels als Regelungs-Vorgang. Z Biol 109:70–80
50. Bösche J, Mallach HJ (1969) Über anatomische und chemischtoxikologische Befunde bei einer tödlichen Vergiftung durch Orphenadrin. Arch Toxicol (Berl) 25:76–82
51. Bonvallet MS, Zbrozyna A (1963) Les commandes reticulaires du système autonome et en particulier de l'innervation sympathique et parasympathique de la pupille. Arch Ital Biol 101:174–207
52. Borgmann H (1967) Das Verhalten des Pupillendurchmessers in Dunkelheit nach verschieden langer Vorbelichtung. Albrecht von Graefes Arch Klin Opthalmol 172:220–228
53. Borgmann H (1972) Grundlagen für eine klinische Pupillographie. II. Abhängigkeit des Pupillendurchmessers in Dunkelheit vom Lebensalter. Albrecht von Graefes Arch Klin Ophthalmol 184:300–308

54. Bosanquet RC, Johnson GJ (1981) Peninsula pupil. Anomaly unique to Newfoundland and Labrador. Arch Ophthalmol 99:1824–1826

55. Bouma H (1965) Receptive systems mediating certain light reaction of the pupil of the human eye. Thesis, Eindhoven

56. Bovino JA, Burton TC (1980) Measurement of the relative afferent pupillary defect in retinal detachment. Am J Ophthalmol 90:19–21

57. Bresky RH, Charles S (1969) Pupil motor perimetry. Am J Ophthalmol 68:108–112

58. Bronster DJ, Rudolph SH, Shanzer S (1983) Pupillar light-near dissociation in cranial arteritis. Neuroophthalmology 3:65–70

59. Brooks B (1956) An intracellular study of the action of the repetitiv nerve volleys and of botulinum toxin on miniature endplate potentials. J Physiol 134:264–277

60. Bürki E (1981) Ophthalmologische Befunde bei der neuralen Muskelatrophie. Klin Montasbl Augenheilkd 179:94–96

61. Bütikofer R, Aubert R (1978) Electronics of contact lens pupillography—A method for binocular stimulating and recording of the pupillary reflex of noncollaborating subjects. Med Biol Eng Comput 16:39–44

62. Bumke O (1903) Ein neues Pupillometer. Münch Med Wochenschr 50:1343–1344

63. Bumke O (1911) Die Pupillenstörungen bei Geistes- und Nervenkrankheiten. Fischer, Jena

64. Bumke O, Krapf E (1936) Vergiftungen durch anorganische und organische sowie durch pflanzliche, tierische und bakterielle Gifte. In: Bumke O, Foerster O (Hrsg) Handbuch der Neurologie, B 13. Springer, Berlin

65. Byrnes DP (1979) Head injury and the dilated pupil. Am Surg 45:139–143

66. Campbell FW, Gregory AH (1960) Effect of size of pupil on visual acuity. Nature 187:1121–1123

67. Carlson VR (1957) Individual pupillary reactions to certain centrally acting drugs in man. J Pharmacol Exp Ther 121:501–506

68. Carpenter MB, Peter Ph (1970) Accessory oculomotor nuclei in the monkey. J Hirnforsch 12:405–418

69. Cassady JR, Light A (1957) Familial persistent pupillary membranes. Arch Ophthalmol 58:438–448

70. Castenholz A (1968) Eine neue Methode zur Beobachtung und Registrierung der Pupillenbewegungen (Pupillo-Kymographie) im Infrarotlicht. Albert von Graefes Arch Klin Ophthalmol 175:100–110

71. Cherington M (1974) Botulism. Arch Neurol 30:432–437

72. Cibis GW, Campos EC, Aulhorn E (1975) Pupillary hemiakinesia in suprageniculte lesions. Arch Ophtalmol 93:1322–1327

73. Cogan DG (1941) Am J Ophthalmol 24:1431–1433

74. Cohen DN, Zakov ZN, Salanga VD, Dohn DF (1975) Raeder's paratrigeminal syndrome. Am J Ophthalmol 79:1044–1049

75. Crosby EC, Henderson JW (1948) The mammalian midbrain and isthmus regions. II. Fiber connection of the superior colliculus. B. Pathways concerned in automatic eye movements. J Comp Neurol 88:53–91

76. Crosby EC, Humphrey T, Lauer EW (1962) Correlative anatomy of the nervous systeme. MacMillan, New York

77. Cross HE, Maumenee AE (1973) Progressive spontaneous dissolution of the iris. Surv Opthalmol 18:186–199

78. Cüppers C (1951) Eine neue Methode zur stetigen Registrierung der konsensuellen Pupillenreaktion. Klin Monatsbl Augenheilkd 119:411–417

79. Currie J, Lessell S (1984) Tonic pupil with giant cell arteritis. Br J Ophthalmol 68:135–138

80. Czarnecki JSC, Thompson HS (1978) The iris sphincter in aberrant regeneration of the third nerve. Arch Ophthalmol 96:1606–1610

81. Daum KM, Fry GA (1981) The component of physiological pupilary unrest correlated with respiration. Am J Optom Physiol Optics. 58:831–840

82. Davidson ST (1973) Report of ocular adverse reactions. Trans Ophthalmol Soc UK 93:495–510

83. Dekking HM (1933) Infrarot-Photographie des Auges. Albrecht von Graefes Arch Klin Ophthalmol 130:373–374

84. Delong SL, Poley BJ, McFarlane Jr (1965) Ocular changes associated with long term chlorpromazine therapy. Arch Ophthalmol 73:611–617

85. Dieterich CE (1973) Die Feinstruktur von M. sphincter und dilatator und ihre Innervation in der menschlichen Iris. In:

Dodt E, Schrader KE (Hrsg) Die normale und gie gestörte Pupillenbewegung. Bermann, München

86. Doesschate J Ten, Alpern M (1965) Response of the pupil to steady-state retinal illumination: Contribution by cones. Science 149:989–991

87. Drance SM (1972) Some factors in the production of the low-tension glaucoma. Br J Ophthalmol 56:229–242

88. Drischel H (1957) Dynamik des Lichtreflexes der menschlichen Pupille. I. Der normale Reflexablauf nach kurzdauernder Belichtung und seine Variabilität Pflügers Arch Ges Physiol 264:148–168

89. Duke-Elder S (1971) System of ophthalmology, vol XII. Kimpton, London

90. Engelking E (1922) Vergleichende Untersuchungen über die Pupillenreaktion bei der angeborenen totalen Farbenblindheit. Klin Monatsbl Augenheilkd 69:177–188

91. Ehinger B (1971) A comparative study of the adrenergic nerves to the anterior eye segment of some primates. Z Zellforsch 116:157–177

92. Ekbom K (1970) A clinical comparison of cluster headache and migraine. Acta Neurol Scand [Suppl 41] 46:1–41

93. Ellis CJK (1979) The afferent pupillary defect in acute optic neuritis. J Neurol Neurosurg Psychiatry 42:1008–1017

94. Ernest JT (1972) Prostaglandins—a missing link? Am J Ophthalmol 74:992–993

95. Fisher CM (1980) Oval pupils. Arch Neurol 37:502–503

96. Fison PN, Garlich DJ, Smith SE (1979) Assessment of unilateral afferent pupillary defects by pupillography. Br J Ophthalmol 63:195–199

97. Flynn JT, Kazarian E, Barricks M (1981) Paradoxical pupil in congenital achromatopsia. Int Ophthalmol Clin 3:91–96

98. Fraunfelder FT (1976) Drug-induced ocular side effects and drug interactions. Lea & Febiger, Philadelphia

99. Freeman MI, Burde RM, Gay AJ (1965) A case of true paradoxical pupillary reaction. Arch Ophthalmol 75:740–741

100. Frydrychowicz G, Harms H (1940) Das pupillomotorische Perimeter. Ber Dtsch Ophthalmol Ges 53:326–329

101. Fugate JM (1954) A masking technique for isolating the pupillary response to focused light. J Opt Soc Am 44:771–779

102. Gabrielides AJ (1952) La dilatateur pupille chez le lapin albinos. Bull Soc Héllenique Opthalmol 19:39

103. Gadoth N, Schlaen N, Maschkowski D, Bechar M (1983) The pupil cycle time in familiar dysautonomia. Metab Pediatr System Ophthalmol 7:131–134

104. Gang K (1945) Psychosomatical factors in the control of pupillary movements. J Clin. Psychopathol (Washington) 6:461–472

105. Gangitano JL, Keltner JL (1980) Abnormalities of the pupil and visual-evoked potential in quinine-amblyopia. Am J Ophthalmol 89:425–430

106. Giles CL, Henderson JW (1958) Horner's syndrome. An analysis of 216 cases. Am J Ophthalmol 46:289–296

107. Gitelson S (1967) Methaqualone-meprobamate poisoning. JAMA 201:977–979

108. Glaser JS (1978) Neuro-ophthalmology. Harper & Row, Hagerstown

109. Gobiet W (1980) Grundlagen der neurologischen Intensivmedizin. Springer, Berlin

110. Godtfredsen E, Gederman N (1965) Diagnostic and prognostic roles of ophthalmoneurologic signs and symptoms in malignant nasopharyngeal tumors. Am J Ophthalmol 59:1063–1069

111. Godwin-Austen RB, Lind NA, Turner P (1969) Mydriatic responses to sympathomimetic amines in patients treated with L-dopa. Lancet 2:13

112. Goldberg ME, Johnson HH (1962) Autonomic ganglion activity and acute toxicologic effects of N, N, N', N'-tetramethyl-1,3 butanediamine and triethyleneadiamine, two foam catalyst amines. Toxicol Appl Pharmacol 4:522–545

113. Goldhammer Y (1977) Paradoxical pupillary light reaction. In: Smith JL (ed) Neuro-ophthalmology update. Masson, New York

114. Gomes B (1943) External ophthalmoplegia from crotal (snake) poison. Ophthalmos 3:187–194

115. Goodman LS, Gilman A (1965) The pharmacological basis of therapeutics, 3rd edn. Macmillan, New York

116. Grant WM (1974) Toxicology of the eye. 2nd edn. Thomas, Springfield

117. Green DG, Maaseidvaag F (1967) Closed circuit television pupillometer. J Opt Soc Am 57:830

118. Greenwald MJ, Folk ER (1983) Afferent pupillary defects in ambylopia. J Pediatr Ophthalmol Strabism 20:63–67

Dodt E, Schrader KE (Hrsg) Die normale und gie gestörte Pupillenbewegung. Bermann, München

86. Doesschate J Ten, Alpern M (1965) Response of the pupil to steady-state retinal illumination: Contribution by cones. Science 149:989–991

87. Drance SM (1972) Some factors in the production of the low-tension glaucoma. Br J Ophthalmol 56:229–242

88. Drischel H (1957) Dynamik des Lichtreflexes der menschlichen Pupille. I. Der normale Reflexablauf nach kurzdauernder Belichtung und seine Variabilität Pflügers Arch Ges Physiol 264:148–168

89. Duke-Elder S (1971) System of ophthalmology, vol XII. Kimpton, London

90. Engelking E (1922) Vergleichende Untersuchungen über die Pupillenreaktion bei der angeborenen totalen Farbenblindheit. Klin Monatsbl Augenheilkd 69:177–188

91. Ehinger B (1971) A comparative study of the adrenergic nerves to the anterior eye segment of some primates. Z Zellforsch 116:157–177

92. Ekbom K (1970) A clinical comparison of cluster headache and migraine. Acta Neurol Scand [Suppl 41] 46:1–41

93. Ellis CJK (1979) The afferent pupillary defect in acute optic neuritis. J Neurol Neurosurg Psychiatry 42:1008–1017

94. Ernest JT (1972) Prostaglandins—a missing link? Am J Ophthalmol 74:992–993

95. Fisher CM (1980) Oval pupils. Arch Neurol 37:502–503

96. Fison PN, Garlich DJ, Smith SE (1979) Assessment of unilateral afferent pupillary defects by pupillography. Br J Ophthalmol 63:195–199

97. Flynn JT, Kazarian E, Barricks M (1981) Paradoxical pupil in congenital achromatopsia. Int Ophthalmol Clin 3:91–96

98. Fraunfelder FT (1976) Drug-induced ocular side effects and drug interactions. Lea & Febiger, Philadelphia

99. Freeman MI, Burde RM, Gay AJ (1965) A case of true paradoxical pupillary reaction. Arch Ophthalmol 75:740–741

00. Frydrychowicz G, Harms H (1940) Das pupillomotorische Perimeter. Ber Dtsch Ophthalmol Ges 53:326–329

01. Fugate JM (1954) A masking technique for isolating the pupillary response to focused light. J Opt Soc Am 44:771–779

02. Gabrielides AJ (1952) La dilatateur pupille chez le lapin albinos. Bull Soc Héllenique Opthalmol 19:39

135. Hepler RS (1977) Adie's tonic pupil. Trans Am Acad Oph-
     thalmol Otolaryngol 83:843–846
136. Hepler RS, Frank IM, Ungerleider J Th (1972) Pupillary con-
     striction after marihuana smoking. Am J Ophthalmol
     74:1185–1190
137. Herxheimer A (1958) A comparison of some atropine-like
     drugs in man, with particular referene to their end-organ spe-
     cifity. Br J Pharmacol 13:184–192
138. Hess C von (1915) Das Differential-Pupilloskop. Arch
     Augenheilkd 80:213–228
139. Hess C von (1929) Pupille. In: Bethe et al (Hrsg) Handbuch
     der normalen und der pathologischen Physiologie. Recep-
     tionsorgane II. Springer, Berlin
140. Hornung J (1966) Über die Bewegungen der menschlichen
     Pupille nach einer sprungartigen Änderung der Reizlichtin-
     tensität. Pflügers Arch Ges Physiol 287:29–40
141. Hunt WE, Meagher JN, Gefever HE, Freman W (1961) Pain-
     ful ophthalmoplegia, its relation to indolent inflammation of
     cavernous sinus. Neurology 11:56–62
142. Ishikawa S, Naito M, Inaba K (1970) A new videopupil-
     lography. Ophthalmologica 160:248–259
143. Jammes JL (1980) Fixed dilated pupils in petit mal attacks.
     Neuro-Ophthalmology 1:155–159
144. Jampel RS (1959) Representation of the near response on the
     cerebral cortex of the macaque. Am J Ophthalmol 48:573–
     582
145. Jarett WH (1967) Horner's syndrome with geniculate zoster.
     Am J Ophthalmol 63:326–330
146. Jensen W (1976) Die Fernsehbildanalyse. Ein Meßverfahren
     zur objektiven Perimetrie. Albrecht von Graefes Arch Klin
     Ophthalmol 201:183–191
147. Johnson FA, Buren HC van (1962) Abstinence syndrome fol-
     lowing glutethimide intoxication. JAMA 180:1024–1027
148. Kase M, Nagata R, Yoshida A, Hanada I (1984) Pupillary light
     reflex in amblyopia. Invest Ophthalmol Vis Sci 25:467–471
149. Keltner JL, Swisher CN, Gay AJ (1975) Myotonic pupils in
     Charcot-Marie-Tooth disease. Arch Ophthalmol 93:1141–
     1148
150. Kern R (1970) Die adrenergischen Rezeptoren der intraocu-
     lären Muskeln des Menschen. Albrecht von Graefes Arch
     Klin Ophthalmol 180:231–248

151. Kerr FW, Hollowell OW (1964) Location of pupillomotor and accommodation fibers in the oculomotor nerve: Experimental observation on paralytic mydriasis. J Neurol Neurosurg Psychiatry 27:473–481
152. Kestenbaum A (1946) Clinical methods of neuro-ophthalmological examination. Grune & Stratton, New York
153. Keulen-De Vos HCJ, Rij GW, Renardel de Lavalette JCG, Jansen JTG (1983) Effect of indomethacin in preventing surgically induced miosis. Br J Ophthalmol 67:94–96
154. Koerner F, Teuber H-L (1973) Visual field defects of the missile injuries to the geniculo-striate pathways in man. Exp Brain Res 18:88–113
155. Kumnick LS (1956) Aging and the latency and duration of pupil constriction in response to light and sound stimuli. J Gerontol 11:391–396
156. Kyrieleis W (1951) Pupillotonie und Adie-Syndrom. Marhold, Berlin
157. Laties AM, Jacobowitz D (1966) A histochemical study of the adrenergic and cholinergic innervation of the anterior segment of the rabbit eye. Invest Ophthalmol 3:592–600
158. Lauber H (1973) Die Wirkung von Psychopharmaka auf die menschliche Pupille. In: Dodt E, Schrader KE (Hrsg) Die normale und die gestörte Pupillenbewegung. Bergmann, München
159. Leinhos R (1959) Die Altersabhängigkeit des Augenpupillendurchmessers. Optik 16:669–671
160. Lemmingson W, Riethe P (1958) Beobachtungen bei Dysgenesis mesodermalis corneae et iridis in Kombination mit Oligodontie. Klin Monatsbl Augenheilkd 133:887–891
161. Levatin P (1959) Pupillary escape in disease of the retina or optic nerve. Arch Ophthalmol 62:768–779
162. Levin M (1960) Eye disturbances in bromide intoxication. Am J Ophthalmol 50:478–483
163. Liempt JAM van, Vriend JA de (1940) Pupillenmessungen bei monochromatischem Licht. Physica 7:961–969
164. Loewenfeld IE (1958) Mechanisms of reflex dilatation of the pupil. Doc Ophthalmol 12:185–448
165. Loewenfeld IE (1973) Supra-spinale Hemmung. Mechanismus und geschichtliche Entwicklung. In: Dodt E, Schrader KE (Hrsg) Die normale und die gestörte Pupillenbewegung. Bergmann, München

166. Loewenfeld IE (1977) "Simple central" anisocoria: A common condition, seldom recognized. Trans Am Acad Ophthalmol Otolaryngol 83:832–839
167. Loewenfeld IE (1979) Pupillary changes related to age. In: Thompson HS (ed) Topics in neuro-ophthalmology. Williams & Wilkins, Baltimore
168. Loewenfeld IE, Thompson HS (1967) The tonic pupil: a re-evaluation. Am Ophthalmol 63:46–87
169. Lowenstein O (1927) Über die sogenannte paradoxe Lichtreaktion der Pupille. Monatsschr Psychiatr Neurol 66:148–167
170. Lowenstein O (1954) Clinical pupillary symptoms in lesion of the optic nerve, optic chiasm and optic tract. Arch Ophthalmol 52:385–403
171. Lowenstein O, Feinberg R, Loewenfeld IE (1963) Pupillary movements during acute and chronic fatigue: A new test for the objective evaluation of tiredness. Invest Ophthalmol 2:138–157
172. Lowenstein O, Friedman ED (1942) Pupillographic studies. I. The present state of pupillography its method and diagnostic significance. Arch Ophthalmol (NY) 27:969–993
173. Lowenstein O, Kawabata H, loewenfeld IE (1964) The pupil as indicator of retinal activity. Am J Ophthalmol 57:569–596
174. Lowenstein O, Loewenfeld IE (1950) Role of sympathetic and parasympathetic system in reflex dilatation of the pupil. Arch Neurol Psychiatry (Chicago) 64:313–340
175. Lowenstein O, Loewenfeld IE (1950) Mutual role of sympathetic and parasympathetic in shaping of the pupillary reflex to light. Arch Neurol Psychiatry (Chicago) 64:341–377
176. Lowenstein O, Loewenfeld IE (1959) Scotopic and photopic thresholds of the pupillary light reflex in normal man. Am J Ophthalmol 48:87–98
177. Lowenstein O, Loewenfeld IE (1958) Electronic pupillography. A new instrument and some clinical applications. Arch Ophthalmol 59:352–363
178. Lowenstein O, Westphal A (1933) Experimentelle und Klinische Studien zur Physiologie und Pathologie der Pupillenbewegungen. Karger, Berlin
179. Lubech MJ (1971) Effects of drugs on ocular muscles. Int Ophthalmol Clin 11(2):35–62
180. Luckiesh M, Moos FK (1934) Area and brightness of stimulus

related to the pupillary light reflex. J Opt Soc Am 24:130–134

181. Lucy DD, Allen MW van, Thompson HS (1967) Holms-Adie syndrome with segmental hypohidrosis. Neurology 17:763–769

182. Machemer H (1933) Eine kinematographische Methode zur Pupillenmessung und Registrierung der Irisbewegung. Klin Monatsbl Augenheilkd 19:302–316

183. Magoun HW, Atlas D, Hare WK, Ranson SW (1936) The afferent path of the pupillary light reflex in the monkey. Brain 59:234–249

184. Marg E, Morgan MW Jr (1949) The pupillary near reflex. The relation of pupillary diameter to accommodation and various components of convergence. Am J Optom Physiol Opt 26:183–189

185. Marg E, Morgan MW (1950) Further investigation of the pupillary near reflex. Am J Optom Physiol Opt 27:217–225

186. Maloney WF, Younge BR, Moyer NJ (1980) Evaluation of the causes and accuracy of pharmacologic localisation in Horner's syndrome. Am J Ophthalmol 90:394–402

187. Martin NR (1967) Opioid antagonists. Pharmacol Rev 19:463–506

188. Matthes K (1941) Über die Registrierung von Bewegungsvorgängen mit dem lichtelektrischen Reflexionsmesser. Klin Wochenschr 20:295–297

189. McCrary JA (1977) Light reflex anatomy and the afferent pupil defect. Trans Am Acad Ophthalmol Otolaryngol 83:820–826

190. McKissock W, Richardson A, Bloom WH (1960) Subdural haematoma. Lancet 1:1365–1369

191. McKissock W, Taylor JC, Bloom WH, Till K (1960) Extradural haematoma. Lancet 2:167–172

192. McNealy DE, Plum F (1962) Brainstem dysfunction with supratentorial mass lesions. Arch Neurol 7:10–32

193. Memon MY, Paine KWE (1971) Direct injury of the oculomotor nerve in cranio cerebral trauma. J Neurosurg 35:461–464

194. Mertz M, Roggenkämper P (1973) Ein bildanaltisches Verfahren zur Messung der Pupillengröße. In: Dodt E, Schrader KE (Hrsg) Die normale und die gestörte Pupillenbewegung. Bergmann, München

195. Meyer BC (1947) Incidence of anisocoria and difference in

size of palpebral fissures in 500 normal subjects. Arch Neurol
Psychiatry (Chicago) 57:464–468

196. Mifka P (1968) Die Augensymptomatik bei den frischen
Schädel-Hirnverletzungen. de Gruyter, Berlin

197. Miller RW, Fraumeni JF Jr, Manning MD (1964) Association
of Wilm's tumor with aniridia, hemihypertrophy and other
congenital malformations. N Engl J Med 270:922–927

198. Miller SD, Thompson HS (1978) Pupil cycle time in optic
neuritis. Am J Ophthalmol 85:635–642

199. Moeschling S (1964) Klinik und Therapie der Vergiftungen.
Thieme, Stuttgart

200. Montgomery J (1959) Two cases of ophthalmoplegia due to
berg adder bite. Cent Afr J Med 5:173

201. Moses RA (1970) Adler's physiology of the eye. Mosby, St.
Louis

202. Müller-Jensen A (1978) Untersuchung zur Pupillen-Lich-
treflex-Dynamik   mittels   Infrarot-Reflexpupillographie.
Fortschr Med 96:27–31

203. Müller-Jensen A, Hagenah R (1976) Untersuchungen zur
Variabilität des phasischen Pupillenlichtreflexes. J Neurol
212:123–132

204. Müller-Jensen A, Hagenah R (1978) Simultaneous recording
of pupillary hippus and EEG. J Neurol 217:213–218

205. Müller-Jensen A, Hagenah R, Igloffstein J (1976) Paradoxe
Lichtreaktion der Pupille. J Neurol 212:101–106

206. Müller-Jensen A, Hellner KA (1977) Die Bedeutung hemi-
anopischer Pupillenlichtreaktion für die Beurteilung der ho-
monymen Hemianopsie. Zentralbl Ges Neurol Psychiatrie
218:282

207. Müller-Jensen K, Albert HH von, Rossi U (1966) Paradoxe
Pupillenreaktion nach operativem Eingriff im Bereich der
Fissura orbitalis cerebralis. Klin Monatsbl Augenheilkd
149:50–57

208. Naumann GOH (1980) Pathologie des Auges. Springer,
Berlin Heidelberg New York

209. O'Connor M, Eustace P (1983) Tonic pupil and lateral rectus
palsy following dental anaesthesia. Neuroophthalmol 3:205–
208

210. Olsen Th, Jakobsen J (1984) Abnormal pupillary function in
the third nerve regeneration (the pseudo-Argyll-Robertson
pupil). Acta Ophthalmol 62:163–167

211. Pant SS, Benton JW, Dodge PR (1966) Unilateral pupillary

dilatation during and immediately following seizures. Neurology (Minneap) 16:837–840

212. Patel H, Crichton JU (1968) Neurological hazards of diphenylhydantoin in childhood. J Pediatr 73:676–684

213. Payne JW, Adamkiewicz J Jr (1969) Unilateral internal ophthalmoplegia with intracranial aneurysm. Am J Ophthalmol 68:349–352

214. Pelêska M (1958) A pupillograph based on an infrared light convertor. Csl Ophthalmol 14:399–410

215. Petajan JH, Danforth RC, D'Allesio DD, Lucas GL (1965) Progressive sudomotor denervation and Adie's syndrome. Neurology 15:172–175

216. Petersen P (1956) Die Pupillographie und das Pupillogramm. Eine methodologische Studie. Acta Physiol Scand [Suppl] 37:125

217. Pevehouse BC, Bloom WH, McKissock W (1960) Ophthalmologic aspects of diagnosis and localisation of subdural hematoma: An analysis of 389 cases and review of the literature. Neurology 10:1037–1041

218. Pfenninger E, Kilian J, Schleinzer W (1982) Differential diagnose des Leitsymptoms "Pupillenveränderung". Klinikarzt 11:1188–1201

219. Portnoy JZ, Thompson HS, Lennarson L, Corbett JO (1983) Pupillary defects in amblyopia. Am J Ophthalmol 96:690–614

220. Ranson SW, Magoun HW (1933) The central path of the pupilloconstrictor reflex in response to light. Arch Neurol Psychiatry (Chicago) 30:1193–1204

221. Rauber-Kopsch (1940) Lehrbuch und Atlas der Anatomie des Menschen, Bd III. Thieme, Leipzig

222. Redslob E (1953) Le dilatateur de la pupille. Ann Ocul 186:289–311

223. Reeves P (1918) Rate of pupillary dilatation and contraction. Psychol Rev 25:330–340

224. Reid HA (1968) Snakebite in the tropics. Br Med J 3:359–362

225. Renard G (1947) La synergie pupillaire á la convergence. Rev Otoneuroophthalmol 19:240–242

226. Reuther R, Alexandridis E, Krastel H (1981) Pupillenreflexstörungen bei Infarkten der Arteria cerebri posterior. I. Pupillometrischer Nachweis. Arch Psychiatr Nervenkr 229:249–257

227. Reuther R, Krastel H, Alexandridis E (1981) Pupillen-

störungen bei Infarkten der Arteria cerebri posterior. II. Pupillometrischer Nachweis von Parazentralskotomen. Arch Psychiatr Nervenkr 229;259–266

228. Richardson KC (1964) The fine structure of the albino rabbit iris with special reference to the identification of adrenergic and cholinergic nerves and nerve endings in its instrinsic muscles. Am J Anat 114:173–205

229. Ridley H (1944) Snake venom ophthalmia. Br J Ophthalmol 28:568

230. Rieger H (1973) Zur Ätiologie der Pupillotonie. In: Dodt E, Schrader KE (Hrsg) Die normale und die gestörte Pupillenbewegung. Bergmann, München

231. Riley FC, Moyer NJ (1970) Experimental Horner's syndrome. A pupillographic evaluation of guanethidine-induced adrenergic blockade in humans. Am J Ophthalmol 69:442–447

232. Rohen JW (1951) Der Bau der Regenbogenhaut beim Menschen und einigen Säugern. Morphol Jahrb 91:140–181

233. Rohen JW (1964) Das Auge und seine Hilfsorgane. In: Bargmann W (Hrsg) Handbuch der mikroskopischen Anatomie des Menschen, B III/4. Springer, Berlin Göttingen Heidelberg New York

234. Ross AT (1958) Progressive selective sudomotor denervation. Neurology (Minneap) 8:809–811

235. Rother P, Leutert G (1966) Über den Alterswandel der menschlichen Iris. Albrecht von Graefes Arch Klin Ophthalmol 170:323–331

236. Ruprecht KW, Naumann GOH (1978) Aniridie und Wilms-Tumor. Ber Dtsch Ophthalmol Ges 75:588–590

237. Sachsenweger R (1977) Neuroophthalmologie. Thieme, Stuttgart

238. Safran AB, Walser A, Roth A, Gauthier G (1981) Influence of central depressant drugs on pupil funktion: An evaluation with the pupils cycle induction test. Ophthalmologica 183:214–219

239. Saladin JJ (1978) Television pupillometry via digital time processing. Invest Ophthalmol 17:702–705

240. Sander E (1929) Über quantitative Messung der Pupillenreaktion und einen in der Praxis hierfür geeigneten einfachen Apparat. Klin Monatsbl Augenheilkd 83:318–322

241. Sattler CH (1932) Augenveränderungen bei Intoxikationen. In: Kurzes Handbuch der Ophthalmologie, B 7. Springer, Berlin

242. Schäfer WD, Leinwand B (1973) Die Bedeutung des Cocain-Adrenalin-Testes beim Hornerschen Symptomenkomplex. In: Dodt E, Schrader KE (Hrsg) Die normale und die gestörte Pupillenbewegung. Bergmann, München

243. Schäfer WD, Richter G (1972) Die Bedeutung des Mecholyl-Testes für die Diagnose der Pupillotonie. Ber Dtsch Ophthalmol Ges 71:554–557

244. Schaeppi U, Koella WP (1964) Innervation of cat iris dilator. Am J Physiol 207:1411–1416

245. Schirmer O (1897) Untersuchungen zur Pathologie der Pupillenweite und der centripetalen Pupillarfasern. Albrecht von Graefes Arch Klin Ophthalmol 44:358–403

246. Schlesinger E (1913) Über den Stellenwert der Pupillenreaktion und die Ausdehnung der pupillomotorischen Bezirke der Retina. Untersuchungen aufgrund einer neuen Methodik. Dtsch Med Wochenschr 31:163–166

247. Schrader KE (1969) Schädigungen des vorderen Augenabschnittes durch Medikamente. Ophthalmologica 158:218–231

248. Schweitzer H (1952) Tödliche Saponinvergiftung durch Genuß von Roßkastanien. Med Klinik 683–685

249. Schweitzer NMJ (1956) Treshold measurements on the light reflex of the pupil in the dark adapted eye. Doc Ophthalmol 10:1–78

250. Simon RD (1963) Parathion poisoning. A case report. Am J Dis Child 105:527

251. Smagghe G (1967) Incidents oculaires par la tetramethylbutanediamine. Arch Mal Prof 28:457–459

252. Smith SA, Smith SE (1980) Contraction anisocoria: nasal versus temporal illumination. Br J Ophthalmol 64:933–934

253. Slooter J, Norren D van (1980) Visual acuity measured with pupil responses to checkerboard stimuli. Invest Ophthalmol Visual Sci 19:105–108

254. Sondermann R (1934) Beitrag zur Kenntnis der Irisentwicklung. Albrecht von Graefes Arch Klin Ophthalmol 133:67–74

255. Spiers ASD, Calne OB, Fayers PM (1970) Miosis during L-dopa therapy. Br Med J 2:639–640

256. Spring KH, Stiles WS (1948) Variation of pupil size with

change in the angle at which the light stimulus strikes the retina. Br J Ophthalmol 32:340–346

257. Staflova J (1969) A comparative study of the adrenergic inner-vation of the iris and ciliary structures in 18 species in phylo-genesis. J Morphol 128:387–401

258. Stark L (1959) Stability, oscillation and noise in the human pupil servomechanism. Proc IRE 47:1925–1939

259. Stark L, Shermann PM (1957) A servoanalytic study of con-sensual pupil reflex to light. J Neurophysiol 20:17–26

260. Stegemann J (1961) Regelungsvorgänge am Auge. Beihefte zur Zeitschrift „Regelungstechnik". Regelungsvorgänge in lebenden Wesen. München

261. Sun F, Stark L (1983) Pupillary escape intensified by large pupillary size. Vision Res 23:611–615

262. Sunderland S (1958) The tentorial notch and complications produced by herniations of the brain through that aperture. Br J Surg 45:422–438

263. Sunderland S, Hughes ESR (1946) The pupilloconstrictor pathway and the nerves to the ocular muscles in man. Brain 69:301–309

264. Teping C, Krastel H, Gärtner RL (1981) Kortikale und pupil-lomotorische Antworten auf Umkehrreize. Ber Dtsch Oph-thalmol Ges 78:735–739

265. Thompson HS (1966) Afferent pupillary deects. Am J Oph-thalmol 62:860–873

266. Thompson HS, Menscher JH (1971) Adrenergic mydriasis in Horner's syndrome. Hydroxyamphetamine test for diag-nosis of postganglionic defects. Am J Ophthalmol 72:472–480

267. Thompson HS, Bourgon P, Allen MW van (1979) The tendon reflexes in Adie's syndrom. In: Thompson HS (ed) Neuro-ophthalmology. Williams & Wilkins, Baltimore.

268. Thompson HS, Allen MW van, Noorden GK von (1964) The pupil in myotonic dystrophy. Invest Ophthalmol 3:325–338

269. Thompson HS, Zackon DH, Czarnecki JSC (1983) Tadpole-shaped pupils caused by segmental spasm of the iris dilator muscle. Am J Ophthalmol 96:467–477

270. Trendelenburg W (1920) Ein einfacher Apparat zur genauen Messung des Augenabstandes, der Pupillenweite, der Hornhaut und des Exophthalmus. Klin Monatsbl Augenheilkd 65:527–535

271. Tolle R, Pornsen N (1969) Thymoleptic mydriasis in the course of treatment. In Pharmacopsychiatry 2:86–98

272. Trier HG (1977) Arzneimittelnebenwirkungen auf Refraktion und Akkommodation. In: Hockwin O, Koch HR (Hrsg) Arzneimittelnebenwirkungen am Auge. Fischer, Stuttgart

273. Uhthoff W, Metzger E (1931) Die Sehgifte und die pharmakologische Beeinflussung des Sehens. Handb Norm Pathol Physiol 12:812–833

274. Ukai K, Higashi JT, Ishikawa S (1980) Edge-light pupil oscillation of optic neuritis. Neuro-Ophthalmology 1:33–43

275. Ullman EV, Mossman FD (1950) Glaucoma and orally administered Belladona. Am J Ophthalmol 33:757–762

276. Van de Kraats J, Smith EP, Slooter JA (1977) Objective measurements by the pupil balance method. Doc Ophthalmol 14:213–219

277. Waardenburg PJ (1954) Die Struktur der menschlichen Iris. Z Morphol Anthropol 46:30–46

278. Wagner R (1954) Probleme und Beispiele biologischer Regelung. Stuttgart

279. Walsh FB, Hoyt WF (1969) Clinical neuro-ophthalmology, 3rd edn, vol I and III. Williams & Wilkins, Baltimore

280. Warwick R (1954) The ocular parasympathetic nerve supply and its mesencephalic sources. J Anat 88:71–93

281. Weinstein JM, Gilder JCV, Thompson HS (1980) Pupil cycle time in optic nerve compressions. Am J Ophthalmol 89:263–267

282. Weintraub MJ, Gaasterland D, Woert MH van (1970) Pupillary effects of levodopa therapy. Development of anisocoria in latent Horner's syndrome. N Engl J Med 283:120–123

283. Wernicke G (1883) Über hemianopische Pupillenreaktion. Fortschr Med 1:49–53

284. Wieland T (1968) Poisonous principles of mushrooms of the genus Amanita. Science 159:946–952

285. Wyatt HJ, Musselman JF (1981) Pupillary light reflex in humans: Evidence for an unbalanced pathway from nasal retina, and for signal cancellation in brainstem. Vision Res 21:513–525

286. Yahr MD, Duvoisin RC, Schear MJ, Barett RE, Hoehm MM (1969) Treatment of parkinsonism with levodopa. Arch Neurol 21:343–354

287. Yamazaki A, Ishikawa S (1976) Abnormal pupillary responses in myasthenia gravis. Br J Ophthalmol 60:575–580
288. Yanoff M, Fine Bs (1975) Ocular pathology. Harper & Row, Hagerstown
289. Yoss RE, Moyer NJ, Hollenhorst RW (1978) Pupil size and spontaneous pupillary waves associated with alertness drowsiness and sleep. Neurology 20:545–554
290. Young RSL, Alpern M (1980) Pupil responses to foveal exchange of monochromatic lights. J Opt Soc Am 70:697–706
291. Zihl J (1980) "Blindsight": Improvement of visually guided eye movements by systematic practice in patients with cerebral blindness. Neuropsychologia 18:71–77

Index